Pocket Guide to the

Essentials of
DIAGNOSIS & TREATMENT

a LANGE medical book

D1412242

Pocket Guide to the

Essentials of
DIAGNOSIS & TREATMENT

a LANGE medical book

Lawrence M. Tierney, Jr., MD
Professor of Medicine
University of California, San Francisco
Associate Chief of Medical Service
Veterans Affairs Medical Center
San Francisco, California

With Associate Authors

Sanjay Saint, MD
Robert Wood Johnson Clinic Scholar
University of Washington, Seattle
Chief Medical Resident, 1995–1996
University of California, San Francisco
Veterans Affairs Medical Center
San Francisco, California

Clinton E. Thompson, MD
Long Valley Community Health Clinic
Laytonville, California
Chief Medical Resident, 1990–1991
University of California, San Francisco
Veterans Affairs Medical Center
San Francisco, California

Mary A. Whooley, MD
Fellow, General Internal Medicine
University of California, San Francisco
Chief Medical Resident, 1995–1996
University of California, San Francisco
Veterans Affairs Medical Center
San Francisco, California

APPLETON & LANGE
Stamford, Connecticut

Copyright © 1997 by Appleton & Lange
A Simon & Schuster Company

97 98 99 00 01 / 10 9 8 7 6 5 4 3 2 1

Prentice Hall International (UK) Limited, *London*
Prentice Hall of Australia Pty. Limited, *Sydney*
Prentice Hall Canada, Inc., *Toronto*
Prentice Hall Hispanoamericana, S.A., *Mexico*
Prentice Hall of India Private Limited, *New Delhi*
Prentice Hall of Japan, Inc., *Tokyo*
Simon & Schuster Asia Pte. Ltd., *Singapore*
Editora Prentice Hall do Brasil Ltda., *Rio de Janeiro*
Prentice Hall, *Upper Saddle River, New Jersey*

Library of Congress Catalog Card Number: 97-70188

ISBN 0-8385-3605-0

9 780838 536056

90000

Acquisitions Editor: Shelley Reinhardt
Developmental Editor: Jim Ransom
Production Editor: Jeanmarie M. Roche

PRINTED IN THE UNITED STATES OF AMERICA

To Jim Ransom

Contents

Preface

This is a small volume originating from an idea of Jack Lange, who believed that some of the elements from the larger textbooks in the Appleton & Lange series might make a useful volume for students, residents, and busy practitioners. The reader familiar with *Current Medical Diagnosis & Treatment,* for example, will recognize the "Essentials of Diagnosis" feature, long an important part of *CMDT.* A similar approach was taken here for differential diagnosis and treatment, with the goal being maximum verbal compression. This book is obviously not intended to be an encyclopedia, but the hope is that the information contained herein will be a valuable adjunct and perhaps a memory stimulant to those who use it. Drs. Thompson, Saint, and Whooley were all superb Chief Medical Residents at UCSF and provided the relevance and currency that we hope will make this a valuable addition to any health care provider's library. To reiterate, the idea, as many others, came from Jack Lange, who has contributed so much to the education of so many.

Lawrence M. Tierney, Jr., MD

San Francisco, California
March 1997

1

Cardiovascular Diseases

Aortic Stenosis

- **Essentials of Diagnosis**
  - Causes include congenital bicuspid valve and progressive valvular calcification of normal valves; rheumatic fever rarely if ever causes isolated aortic stenosis
  - Dyspnea, angina, and syncope singly or in any combination; sudden death in less than 5%
  - Weak and delayed carotid pulses; a soft, absent, or paradoxically split S_2; a harsh diamond-shaped systolic ejection murmur to the right of the sternum, often radiating to the neck
  - Electrocardiography shows left ventricular hypertrophy; and x-ray may show calcification in aortic valve
  - Echo-Doppler confirms the diagnosis and estimates the valve area and gradient; cardiac catheterization confirms severity, documents concomitant coronary atherosclerotic disease

- **Differential Diagnosis**
  - Mitral regurgitation
  - Hypertrophic obstructive cardiomyopathy
  - Atrial septal defect
  - Ventricular septal defect
  - Syncope of other causes, eg, ventricular tachycardia

- **Treatment**
  - Any medical therapy can potentially worsen symptoms
  - Surgery is indicated for all symptomatic patients, ideally before heart failure develops
  - Asymptomatic patients considered for surgery if the valve gradient is severe (> 60 mm Hg) or with advanced left ventricular dysfunction
  - Percutaneous balloon valvuloplasty for temporary (6 months) relief of symptoms in poor surgical candidates

1

Aortic Regurgitation

■ Essentials of Diagnosis

- Causes include congenital bicuspid valve, endocarditis, hypertension, rheumatic heart disease, and aortic root diseases (Marfan's syndrome, aortic dissection, ankylosing spondylitis, Reiter's syndrome, and syphilis)
- Acute aortic regurgitation: acute onset of pulmonary edema
- Chronic aortic regurgitation: generally asymptomatic until middle age, when chest pain or symptoms of left heart failure develop
- Reduced first heart sound, wide pulse pressure, water-hammer pulse, subungual capillary pulsations (Quincke's sign), rapid rise and fall of pulse (Corrigan's pulse), and a diastolic murmur over a partially compressed femoral artery (Duroziez' sign).
- Soft, high-pitched, decrescendo diastolic murmur; occasionally, an accompanying apical low-pitched diastolic rumble (Austin Flint murmur) in nonrheumatic patients
- Electrocardiography shows left ventricular hypertrophy, and x-ray shows left ventricular dilation
- Echo-Doppler confirms diagnosis, estimates severity

■ Differential Diagnosis

- Mitral or, rarely, tricuspid stenosis
- Left ventricular failure due to other cause

■ Treatment

- Vasodilators (eg, nifedipine and ACE inhibitors) delay the progression to valve replacement
- In chronic aortic regurgitation, surgery reserved for patients with symptoms of left ventricular dysfunction
- Acute regurgitation caused by aortic dissection or endocarditis requires surgical replacement of the valve

Mitral Stenosis

- ■ Essentials of Diagnosis
  - Caused by rheumatic heart disease
  - Dyspnea, orthopnea, paroxysmal nocturnal dyspnea, even hemoptysis—often precipitated by volume overload (pregnancy, salt load) or tachycardia
  - Crisp S_1, increased P_2, opening snap; these sounds often easier to appreciate than the characteristic low-pitched apical diastolic murmur
  - Right ventricular lift in many; S_1 snap occasionally palpable
  - Electrocardiography shows left atrial abnormality and, commonly, atrial fibrillation; echo-Doppler confirms diagnosis, quantifies severity

- ■ Differential Diagnosis
  - Left ventricular failure due to any cause
  - Mitral valve prolapse (if systolic murmur present)
  - Pulmonary hypertension due to other cause
  - Left atrial myxoma
  - Cor triatriatum (in patients under 30)
  - Tricuspid stenosis

- ■ Treatment
  - Heart failure symptoms may be treated with diuretics and sodium restriction
  - With atrial fibrillation, ventricular rate controlled with digoxin, long-term anticoagulation instituted with warfarin
  - Valvuloplasty or valve replacement in symptomatic patients with mitral orifice of less than 1.2 cm^2
  - Prophylaxis for infective endocarditis

1

Mitral Regurgitation

- **Essentials of Diagnosis**
  - Causes include rheumatic heart disease, myxomatous degeneration, ischemic papillary muscle dysfunction
  - Acute mitral regurgitation: immediate onset of symptoms of pulmonary edema
  - Chronic mitral regurgitation: asymptomatic for years, then exertional dyspnea and fatigue
  - S_1 usually reduced; blowing, high-pitched pansystolic murmur over the apex is characteristic; S_3 common
  - Electrocardiography shows left atrial abnormality and often left ventricular hypertrophy; atrial fibrillation typical in chronic cases
  - Echo-Doppler confirms diagnosis, estimates severity

- **Differential Diagnosis**
  - Aortic stenosis or sclerosis
  - Tricuspid regurgitation
  - Hypertrophic obstructive cardiomyopathy
  - Atrial septal defect
  - Ventricular septal defect

- **Treatment**
  - Acute mitral regurgitation due to endocarditis or ischemia often requires immediate surgical repair
  - Patients with chronic mitral regurgitation require prophylaxis for infective endocarditis; surgical repair for severe symptoms, left ventricular dysfunction not responsive to medical management
  - Mild to moderate symptoms can be treated with diuretics, sodium restriction, and afterload reduction (eg, ACE inhibitors); digoxin controls ventricular response with atrial fibrillation, and warfarin anticoagulation should be given

Pulmonary Stenosis

- **Essentials of Diagnosis**
  - A congenital disorder that causes symptoms only when the stenosis is moderate to severe (ie, transpulmonary valve gradient is > 50 mm Hg)
  - Exertional dyspnea and chest pain due to right ventricular ischemia; sudden death occurs in severe cases
  - Jugular venous distention, parasternal lift, a systolic ejection murmur, and a delayed pulmonary component of S_2
  - Right ventricular hypertrophy on ECG; poststenotic dilation of the main and left pulmonary arteries on chest x-ray
  - Echo-Doppler is diagnostic

- **Differential Diagnosis**
  - Left ventricular failure due to any cause
  - Left-sided valvular disease
  - Primary pulmonary hypertension
  - Chronic pulmonary embolism
  - Sleep apnea
  - COPD
  - Eisenmenger's syndrome

- **Treatment**
  - All patients require endocarditis prophylaxis
  - Symptomatic patients can be treated with percutaneous balloon or surgical valvuloplasty
  - Prognosis for those with mild disease is good

1

Aortic Coarctation

- **Essentials of Diagnosis**
  - Elevated blood pressure in the aortic arch and its branches; reduced pressure distally
  - Lower extremity claudication in young adults is characteristic
  - Systolic blood pressure is higher in the arms than in the legs, but diastolic pressure is similar
  - Femoral pulses are decreased, and pulsatile collaterals may be present in the intercostal areas; a harsh systolic murmur may be heard in the back; aortic insufficiency murmur heard because the bicuspid aortic valve is associated
  - Electrocardiography usually shows left ventricular hypertrophy; chest x-ray may show rib notching inferiorly due to collaterals
  - Echo-Doppler is diagnostic

- **Differential Diagnosis**
  - Essential hypertension
  - Renal artery stenosis
  - Renal parenchymal disease
  - Pheochromocytoma
  - Mineralocorticoid excess
  - Oral contraceptive use
  - Cushing's syndrome

- **Treatment**
  - Surgery is the mainstay of therapy; balloon angioplasty in selected patients
  - All patients require endocarditis prophylaxis even after correction
  - Twenty-five percent of patients remain hypertensive after surgery

Atrial Septal Defect

- ■ Essentials of Diagnosis
  - Patients with small defects are usually asymptomatic and have a normal life span
  - Large shunts cause symptoms by age 40, including exertional dyspnea, fatigue, and palpitations
  - Right ventricular lift, widened and fixed splitting of S_2, and systolic flow murmur in the pulmonary area
  - Electrocardiography may show right ventricular hypertrophy and right axis deviation; complete or incomplete right bundle branch block in 95%
  - Echo-Doppler is diagnostic; radionuclide angiogram estimates the ratio of pulmonary flow to systemic flow (PF:SF)

- ■ Differential Diagnosis
  - Left ventricular failure
  - Left-sided valvular disease
  - Primary pulmonary hypertension
  - Chronic pulmonary embolism
  - Sleep apnea
  - COPD
  - Eisenmenger's syndrome
  - Pulmonary stenosis

- ■ Treatment
  - Small defects do not require surgical correction
  - Surgery is indicated for patients with PF:SF > 2.0
  - Surgery is contraindicated in patients with pulmonary hypertension and right-to-left shunting
  - Endocarditis prophylaxis generally unnecessary

Ventricular Septal Defect

- ■ Essentials of Diagnosis
  - Symptoms depend on the size of the defect and the magnitude of the left-to-right shunt
  - Many congenital ventricular septal defects close spontaneously during childhood
  - Small defects in adults are usually asymptomatic except for complicating endocarditis
  - Large defects usually associated with a loud pansystolic murmur along the left sternal border, a systolic thrill, and a loud P_2
  - Echo-Doppler diagnostic; radionuclide angiogram quantifies the ratio of pulmonary flow to systemic flow (PF:SF)

- ■ Differential Diagnosis
  - Mitral regurgitation
  - Aortic stenosis
  - Cardiomyopathy due to various causes

- ■ Treatment
  - Small shunts in asymptomatic patients may not require surgery
  - Mild dyspnea can be treated with diuretics and preload reduction
  - Large shunts should be repaired to prevent irreversible pulmonary vascular disease
  - Surgery if patient has developed shunt reversal (Eisenmenger's syndrome)
  - Prophylaxis for infective endocarditis

Patent Ductus Arteriosus

- **Essentials of Diagnosis**
  - Caused by failure of closure of embryonic ductus arteriosus, with continuous flow of blood from aorta to pulmonary artery
  - Symptoms are those of left ventricular failure or pulmonary hypertension, but many patients are free of complaints
  - Widened pulse pressure, a loud S_2, and a continuous, rough, "machinery" murmur loudest over the pulmonary area
  - Echo-Doppler helpful, but aortography is the study of choice

- **Differential Diagnosis**

  If patients present with left heart failure:
  - Mitral regurgitation
  - Aortic stenosis
  - Ventricular septal defect

  If pulmonary hypertension dominates the picture, consider:
  - Primary pulmonary hypertension
  - Chronic pulmonary embolism
  - Eisenmenger's syndrome

- **Treatment**
  - Pharmacologic closure in premature infants, using indomethacin or aspirin
  - Surgical closure in patients with large shunts or symptoms; efficacy in the presence of pulmonary hypertension is debated
  - Prophylaxis for infective endocarditis

Tricuspid Stenosis

- **Essentials of Diagnosis**
  - Usually rheumatic in origin; rarely seen in carcinoid heart disease
  - Almost always associated with mitral stenosis when rheumatic
  - Evidence of right-sided failure: hepatomegaly, ascites, peripheral edema, jugular venous distention with prominent *a* wave
  - A diastolic rumbling murmur along the left sternal border, increasing with inspiration
  - Echo-Doppler is diagnostic

- **Differential Diagnosis**
  - Aortic regurgitation
  - Mitral stenosis
  - Pulmonary hypertension due to any cause with right heart failure

- **Treatment**
  - Valve replacement in severe cases
  - Balloon valvuloplasty may prove to be useful in many patients

Tricuspid Regurgitation

- **Essentials of Diagnosis**
  - Causes include infective endocarditis, right ventricular heart failure, carcinoid syndrome, systemic lupus erythematosus, and Ebstein's anomaly
  - Most cases secondary to left-sided heart disease
  - Edema, abdominal discomfort, anorexia; otherwise, symptoms those of associated disease
  - Prominent *v* waves in jugular venous pulse; pulsatile liver, hepatojugular reflux
  - A high-pitched blowing systolic murmur along the left sternal border that increases with inspiration is characteristic
  - Echo-Doppler is diagnostic

- **Differential Diagnosis**
  - Mitral regurgitation
  - Aortic stenosis
  - Pulmonary stenosis
  - Atrial septal defect
  - Ventricular septal defect

- **Treatment**
  - Diuretics and dietary sodium restriction in patients with evidence of fluid overload
  - If symptoms are severe and tricuspid regurgitation is primary, valve repair, valvuloplasty, or removal is preferable to valve replacement

Angina Pectoris

■ **Essentials of Diagnosis**

- Pressure-like episodic precordial chest discomfort, precipitated by exertion or stress, relieved by rest or nitrates
- Generally from atherosclerotic coronary artery obstruction; cigarette smoking, diabetes, hypertension, hypercholesterolemia, and a family history of premature coronary artery disease predispose
- S_3, S_4, mitral murmur, reversed splitting of S_2 may occur transiently with pain
- Electrocardiography usually normal between episodes (or may show evidence of old infarction); 20% have normal tracing with pain
- Electrocardiography with pain shows evidence of ischemia, classically ST depression
- Diagnosis from history and stress tests; confirmed and staged by coronary arteriography

■ **Differential Diagnosis**

- Other coronary disorders (myocardial infarction, unstable angina, vasospasm)
- Tietze's syndrome (costochondritis)
- Intercostal neuropathy, especially caused by herpes zoster
- Cervical radiculopathy
- Peptic ulcer disease
- Esophageal spasm or reflux disease
- Cholecystitis
- Pericarditis
- Pneumothorax
- Pulmonary embolism
- Pneumococcal pneumonia

■ **Treatment**

- Address reversible risk factors (smoking, hypertension, hypercholesterolemia)
- Sublingual nitroglycerin as needed for individual episodes
- Ongoing treatment includes long-acting nitrates, beta-blockers, and calcium channel blockers
- Angioplasty considered in patients with anatomically suitable stenoses who have not benefited from medications
- Bypass grafting for patients with angina refractory to medical therapy, triple vessel disease with decreased left ventricular function, or left main disease

Coronary Vasospasm

- Essentials of Diagnosis
  - Caused by intermittent focal spasm of an otherwise normal coronary artery
  - The chest pain resembles typical angina; often more severe and occurs at rest
  - Typically affects women under 50, occurs in the early morning, and involves the right coronary artery
  - Electrocardiography shows ST elevation
  - Diagnosis can be confirmed by ergonovine challenge during cardiac catheterization

- Differential Diagnosis
  - Typical angina pectoris
  - Myocardial infarction
  - Unstable angina
  - Tietze's syndrome (costochondritis)
  - Cervical radiculopathy
  - Peptic ulcer disease
  - Esophageal spasm or reflux disease
  - Cholecystitis
  - Pericarditis
  - Pneumothorax
  - Pulmonary embolism
  - Pneumococcal pneumonia

- Treatment
  - Nitrates and calcium channel blockers effective acutely
  - Long-acting nitrates and calcium channel blockers are the mainstay of chronic therapy

Unstable Angina

- ■ Essentials of Diagnosis
  - Spectrum of illness between chronic stable angina and acute myocardial infarction
  - Characterized by accelerating or "crescendo" angina, pain at rest, or pain that is less responsive to medications
  - Usually due to atherosclerotic plaque rupture, spasm, hemorrhage, or thrombosis
  - Chest pain resembles typical angina but is more severe and lasts longer (but less than 30 minutes)
  - Electrocardiography shows evidence of ST depression or T wave changes during pain, but normalizes when symptoms abate

- ■ Differential Diagnosis
  - Typical angina pectoris
  - Myocardial infarction
  - Coronary vasospasm
  - Tietze's syndrome (costochondritis)
  - Cervical radiculopathy
  - Peptic ulcer disease
  - Esophageal spasm or reflux disease
  - Cholecystitis
  - Pericarditis
  - Pneumothorax
  - Pulmonary embolism
  - Pneumococcal pneumonia

- ■ Treatment
  - Hospitalization at bed rest, telemetry, and exclusion of myocardial infarction
  - Beta-blockers to keep heart rate and blood pressure in the low-normal range
  - Low-dose aspirin (80–325 mg) should be given on admission and every day thereafter; intravenous heparin is of benefit in patients symptomatic despite above measures
  - Nitroglycerin, either in paste or intravenously
  - Cardiac catheterization and consideration of revascularization in appropriate candidates

Acute Myocardial Infarction

- ■ Essentials of Diagnosis
  - Most commonly due to occlusion of a coronary artery by a thrombus at the site of preexisting atherosclerotic stenosis
  - Prolonged (> 30 minutes) chest pain, associated with shortness of breath, nausea, left arm or neck pain, and diaphoresis; can be painless in diabetics
  - Hypotension, congestive heart failure, ventricular arrhythmias, heart block may complicate
  - Electrocardiography shows ST elevation or depression, symmetric T wave inversion, or evolving Q wave development
  - Cardiac enzymes (troponin, CKMB) elevated in the vast majority
  - Echocardiography reveals new regional wall motion abnormality
  - Non-Q wave infarct usually results from incomplete occlusion or spontaneous lysis and signifies the presence of additional jeopardized myocardium

- ■ Differential Diagnosis
  - Angina pectoris
  - Coronary vasospasm
  - Tietze's syndrome (costochondritis)
  - Cervical radiculopathy
  - Peptic ulcer disease
  - Esophageal spasm or reflux disease
  - Cholecystitis
  - Pericarditis
  - Pneumothorax
  - Pulmonary embolism
  - Pneumococcal pneumonia

- ■ Treatment
  - Hospitalization in a coronary care unit, bed rest, telemetry, oxygen, aspirin, and pain relief for all patients; heparin for many
  - Immediate opening of the occluded vessel by thrombolysis or angioplasty should be considered in selected patients
  - Beta-blockers to keep heart rate and blood pressure in the low-normal range and for survival advantage when given chronically
  - Nitroglycerin for recurrent ischemic pain; also useful for relieving pulmonary congestion and reducing blood pressure
  - ACE inhibitor for those with ejection fractions less than 40%

Atrial Fibrillation

- **Essentials of Diagnosis**
  - The most common chronic arrhythmia
  - Causes include mitral valve disease, hypertensive and ischemic heart disease, dilated cardiomyopathy, alcohol, thyrotoxicosis, pericarditis, cardiac surgery; many are idiopathic ("lone" atrial fibrillation)
  - Complications include precipitation of cardiac failure, arterial embolization
  - Palpitations, shortness of breath, chest pain common
  - Irregularly irregular heart beat, variable intensity S_1, occasional S_3; mitral regurgitation, friction rub in some patients
  - Electrocardiography shows ventricular rate of 80–200 in untreated patients; if associated with an accessory pathway, the ventricular rate can be > 200/min with wide QRS

- **Differential Diagnosis**
  - Multifocal atrial tachycardia
  - Atrial flutter or tachycardia with variable block
  - First 50 beats of ventricular tachycardia (if QRS is wide)

- **Treatment**
  - Control ventricular response with beta-blocker, calcium channel blocker, or digoxin
  - Cardioversion with countershock in unstable patients with acute atrial fibrillation; elective countershock or antiarrhythmic agents in stable patients
  - Chronic warfarin in most patients not cardioverted
  - With elective cardioversion, anticoagulation for 4 weeks prior to and continued for 4 weeks after the procedure

| **Atrial Flutter** | **1** |

- ## Essentials of Diagnosis
  - Especially common in patients with COPD, cardiomyopathy (eg, alcoholic cardiomyopathy)
  - Atrial rate between 250 and 350 beats/min with every second, third, or fourth impulse conducted by the ventricle
  - Patients may be asymptomatic, complain of palpitations, or have evidence of congestive heart failure
  - Flutter *a* waves visible in the neck in occasional patients
  - Electrocardiography shows "saw-tooth" P waves in V_1 and the inferior leads; the ventricular response may be regular or, less commonly, irregular due to variable atrioventricular block

- ## Differential Diagnosis
  With regular ventricular rate:
  - Automatic atrial tachycardia
  - Atrioventricular nodal reentry tachycardia
  - Ventricular tachycardia (after first 50 beats)
  - Sinus tachycardia
  With irregular ventricular rate:
  - Atrial fibrillation
  - Multifocal atrial tachycardia
  - First 50 beats of ventricular tachycardia (if QRS is wide)

- ## Treatment
  - Often spontaneously converts to atrial fibrillation
  - Electrical cardioversion is most reliable and safest therapy
  - Conversion may also be achieved by drugs (short-term class 1a or 1c agents with concomitant administration of an atrioventricular conduction blocker)
  - Routine anticoagulation is unnecessary given the low risk of embolization

Multifocal Atrial Tachycardia

- **Essentials of Diagnosis**
    - Commonly seen in COPD or electrolyte abnormalities (especially hypomagnesemia or hypokalemia)
    - Symptoms are usually those of the underlying disorder, but some may complain of palpitations
    - Irregularly irregular heart rate
    - Electrocardiography shows at least three different P wave morphologies with varying P–P intervals
    - Rate usually between 100 and 140 beats/min; if less than 100 beats/min, the rhythm is referred to as "wandering atrial pacemaker"

- **Differential Diagnosis**
    - Atrial fibrillation
    - Atrial flutter with variable block
    - First 50 beats of ventricular tachycardia (if QRS is wide)

- **Treatment**
    - Treatment of the underlying disorder
    - Verapamil or other atrioventricular node blockers for rate control, though digitalis usually ineffective
    - In refractory cases, atrioventricular nodal ablation with permanent pacing

Paroxysmal Supraventricular Tachycardia (PSVT)

- ■ Essentials of Diagnosis
  - A group of arrhythmias including supraventricular reentrant tachycardia, automatic atrial tachycardia, and junctional tachycardia
  - Attacks usually begin and end abruptly, last seconds to hours
  - Patients often asymptomatic but occasionally complain of palpitations, mild shortness of breath, or chest pain
  - Electrocardiography between attacks normal unless the patient has Wolff-Parkinson-White syndrome
  - Unless aberrant conduction occurs, the QRS complexes are regular and narrow; the location of the P wave helps determine the cause of the PSVT
  - Electrophysiologic study establishes the exact diagnosis

- ■ Differential Diagnosis
  Short RP:
  - Atrioventricular reentrant tachycardia
  - Intra-atrial reentry tachycardia
  Long RP:
  - Atrial tachycardia
  - Atypical atrioventricular nodal reentry tachycardia
  - Permanent junctional reciprocating tachycardia
  No P:
  - Atrioventricular nodal reentry tachycardia

- ■ Treatment
  - Many attacks resolve spontaneously and therefore require no treatment acutely—only prevention if recurrent
  - Treatment of the acute attack includes vagal maneuvers (such as carotid sinus massage), drugs (adenosine, calcium channel blockers, beta-blockers), and synchronized electrical cardioversion
  - Prevention of frequent attacks can be achieved by digoxin, channel blockers, beta-blockers, or procainamide; if drug therapy is unsuccessful, patients should be considered for electrophysiologic studies and ablation of the abnormal current

Ventricular Tachycardia

- ■ Essentials of Diagnosis
  - Defined as three or more consecutive premature ventricular beats; can be either nonsustained (lasting < 30 seconds) or sustained (> 30 seconds)
  - The usual mechanisms are reentry (more common) or automatic focus; may occur spontaneously or in the setting of acute myocardial infarction
  - Common additional causes include acute or chronic myocardial ischemia, cardiomyopathy, electrolyte abnormalities, or drug toxicity (eg, oral antiarrhythmics)
  - Most patients are symptomatic; syncope, palpitations, shortness of breath, and chest pain are common
  - S_1 of variable intensity, S_3 typically present
  - Electrocardiography shows a regular, wide-complex tachycardia (usually between 140 and 220 beats/min); between attacks, the ECG often shows evidence of prior myocardial infarction

- ■ Differential Diagnosis
  - Any cause of supraventricular tachycardia with aberrant conduction (in patients with a history of myocardial infarction or low ejection fraction, ventricular tachycardia is much more likely than supraventricular tachycardia)
  - Atrial flutter with aberrant conduction

- ■ Treatment
  - Acute treatment depends upon whether the patient is stable or unstable
  - If stable: intravenous lidocaine or procainamide can be used initially
  - If unstable (hypotension, congestive heart failure, or angina): immediate synchronized cardioversion
  - For chronic recurrent sustained ventricular tachycardia, suppressive treatment guided by electrophysiologic studies or Holter monitoring is needed
  - Patients not responding to or intolerant of antiarrhythmic therapy should be considered for automatic implantable cardiac defibrillator placement
  - Treatment of recurrent, asymptomatic, nonsustained ventricular tachycardia is controversial

Sudden Cardiac Death

- ### ■ Essentials of Diagnosis
  - Defined as nontraumatic and unexpected death in a previously well patient within 1 hour after symptom onset
  - Sudden cardiac death can be due to cardiac or noncardiac disease
  - The most common cause is due to ventricular fibrillation in the setting of coronary artery disease
  - Ventricular fibrillation—a chaotic ventricular rhythm—is almost always the terminal rhythm
  - Since organized electrical activity and ventricular depolarization do not occur, patients have no pulse or blood pressure

- ### ■ Differential Diagnosis
  Noncardiac causes of sudden death:
  - Pulmonary embolism
  - Asthma
  - Aortic dissection
  - Stroke
  - Anaphylaxis

- ### ■ Treatment
  - If sudden cardiac death occurs in the setting of acute myocardial infarction, long-term management is no different from that of other patients with myocardial infarction
  - In the absence of myocardial infarction, the recurrence rate of sudden cardiac death may be as high as 50% in 2 years; therefore, an aggressive approach (cardiac catheterization, revascularization) to prevent another event is warranted
  - Transient abnormalities—electrolyte abnormalities, digitalis toxicity, pacemaker malfunction—should be sought and corrected
  - In patients without an obvious cause, echocardiography and cardiac catheterization are indicated
  - Electrophysiologic studies or ambulatory electrocardiography is indicated in patients who do not have a cause elucidated by the above evaluation
  - An automatic implantable cardiac defibrillator should be strongly considered if (1) ventricular tachycardia cannot be induced by electrophysiologic studies or (2) ventricular tachycardia cannot be suppressed by antiarrhythmics

Atrioventricular Block

- **Essentials of Diagnosis**
  - Categorized as first, second, or third-degree
  - First-degree block is due to delayed conduction at the level of the atrioventricular node and is characterized by a fixed prolonged (> 0.20 s) PR interval
  - Second-degree block is subdivided into Mobitz I (or Wenckebach) and Mobitz II:
    1. Mobitz I—due to delayed conduction of the atrioventricular node—is characterized by progressive prolongation of the PR interval and decreasing R–R prior to blocked sinus impulse
    2. Mobitz II—due to infranodal conduction system disease—is characterized by fixed PR intervals before a beat is dropped
  - Third-degree block is due to complete block at the level of or below the node; the ECG shows P waves and QRS complexes occurring independently, both at fixed rates
  - Clinical manifestations of third-degree block include chest pain, syncope, and shortness of breath; cannon *a* waves may be present on the neck examination; the first heart sound varies in intensity

- **Differential Diagnosis**
  Causes of first-degree and Mobitz I atrioventricular block:
  - Increased vagal tone
  - Drugs that prolong atrioventricular conduction
  - Intrinsic conduction system disease
  Causes of third-degree and Mobitz II atrioventricular block:
  - Chronic degenerative conduction system disease (Lev's and Lenegre's syndromes)
  - Acute anterior myocardial infarction
  - Acute myocarditis
  - Digitalis toxicity
  - Congenital

- **Treatment**
  - No treatment is required in patients with first-degree atrioventricular block or stable patients with Mobitz I; in unstable patients with Mobitz I block, atropine or temporary pacing is indicated to increase the heart rate
  - Those with Mobitz II or infranodal third-degree atrioventricular block require permanent pacing

Cardiac Failure

- ■ **Essentials of Diagnosis**
  - In systolic dysfunction, the ejection fraction is decreased due to pump failure
  - Causes include coronary artery disease, dilated cardiomyopathy, myocarditis, and late stages of valvular and hypertensive disease
  - In diastolic dysfunction, the ejection fraction tends to be normal and cardiac relaxation and diastolic filling are impaired
  - Causes include ischemia, hypertension, aortic stenosis, hypertrophic cardiomyopathy, restrictive cardiomyopathy (eg, amyloidosis), and small vessel disease, particularly diabetes
  - In most patients, systolic and diastolic dysfunction coexist; however, up to 20% will have isolated diastolic dysfunction
  - Symptoms and signs can result from left-sided failure, right-sided failure, or both
  - Left ventricular failure: orthopnea, paroxysmal nocturnal dyspnea, rales, gallop rhythm; pulmonary venous congestion on chest x-ray
  - Right ventricular failure: fatigue, malaise, elevated venous pressure, hepatomegaly, and dependent edema
  - Diagnosis is confirmed by noninvasive (echocardiography, multigated angiography) or hemodynamic measurements (pulmonary capillary wedge measurement)

- ■ **Differential Diagnosis**
  - Pericardial constriction, nephrotic syndrome, and cirrhosis for biventricular failure
  - Mitral stenosis in right ventricular failure
  - Numerous pulmonary diseases (eg, asthma in left-sided disease)

- ■ **Treatment**
  - Systolic dysfunction: vasodilators (ACE inhibitors or combination of hydralazine and isosorbide dinitrate), digoxin, low-sodium diet, and diuretics; beta-blockers and amiodarone are advocated by some
  - Diastolic dysfunction: a negative inotrope (beta-blocker or calcium channel blocker), low-sodium diet, and diuretics

1

Myocarditis

- ■ Essentials of Diagnosis
  - Focal or diffuse inflammation of the myocardium due to various infections, toxins, drugs, or immunologic reactions; viral infection, particularly with coxsackieviruses, is the most common cause
  - Patients usually present with fever, fatigue, palpitations, chest pain, or symptoms of congestive heart failure, often following an upper respiratory tract infection
  - Physical examination findings include fever, disproportionate tachycardia, or signs of congestive heart failure
  - Electrocardiography may reveal ST–T wave changes or intraventricular conduction delay
  - Echocardiography shows diffusely depressed left ventricular function and, if pericarditis is also present, a pericardial effusion
  - Myocardial biopsy may reveal characteristic inflammation, but the lesion is often focal

- ■ Differential Diagnosis
  - Acute myocardial ischemia or infarction due to coronary artery disease; pneumonia; congestive heart failure due to other causes
  Other infectious causes of myocarditis:
  - Scrub typhus
  - Rocky mountain spotted fever
  - Q fever
  - Chagas' disease
  - Lyme disease
  - AIDS
  - Trichinosis
  - Toxoplasmosis
  - Rheumatic fever

- ■ Treatment
  - Bed rest
  - Specific antimicrobial treatment if an infectious agent can by identified; immunosuppressive therapy is controversial
  - Appropriate treatment of the systolic dysfunction that may develop: vasodilators (ACE inhibitors or combination of hydralazine and isosorbide dinitrate), digoxin, low-sodium diet, and diuretics; beta-blockers and amiodarone are advocated by some

Dilated Cardiomyopathy

■ Essentials of Diagnosis

- A cause of systolic dysfunction, this represents a group of disorders that lead to congestive heart failure
- Symptoms and signs of congestive heart failure: exertional dyspnea, cough, fatigue, paroxysmal nocturnal dyspnea, cardiac enlargement, rales, gallop rhythm, elevated venous pressure, hepatomegaly, and dependent edema
- Electrocardiography may show nonspecific repolarization abnormalities and atrial or ventricular ectopy but is not diagnostic
- Echocardiography reveals depressed contractile function and cardiomegaly
- Cardiac catheterization is useful to exclude ischemia as a cause

■ Differential Diagnosis

Causes of dilated cardiomyopathy:
- Alcohol
- Post viral myocarditis
- Sarcoidosis
- Postpartum
- Doxorubicin toxicity
- Endocrinopathies (thyroid disease, acromegaly, pheochromocytoma)
- Hemochromatosis
- Idiopathic

■ Treatment

- Treat the underlying disorder if it can be discerned
- Patients should abstain from alcohol if this is thought to play a role
- Routine management of systolic dysfunction includes vasodilators (ACE inhibitors or combination of hydralazine and isosorbide dinitrate); digoxin; low-sodium diet, and diuretics
- Beta-blockers and amiodarone are advocated by some

Hypertrophic Obstructive Cardiomyopathy (HOCM)

- ■ Essentials of Diagnosis
  - In this disorder, inappropriate myocardial hypertrophy (usually of the interventricular septum) occurs, characteristically causing obstruction to left ventricular outflow just below the aortic valve
  - In young adults, the disorder occurs sporadically or is inherited in an autosomal dominant pattern; many elderly patients have a history of hypertension
  - Obstruction worsened by factors that increase left ventricular contractility or decrease left ventricular filling
  - The most common symptoms are dyspnea, chest pain, and syncope
  - Examination shows sustained, bifid, or, rarely, trifid apical impulse, S_4, and a systolic murmur
  - Electrocardiography shows left ventricular hypertrophy and exaggerated septal Q waves which may suggest myocardial infarction
  - Echocardiography is diagnostic and shows left ventricular hypertrophy—which may be asymmetric—and enhanced contractility with evidence of dynamic obstruction

- ■ Differential Diagnosis
  - Hypertensive heart disease
  - Restrictive cardiomyopathy (eg, amyloidosis)
  - Aortic stenosis
  - Ischemic heart disease

- ■ Treatment
  - Beta-blockers are the initial drug of choice in symptomatic patients, especially those with evidence of dynamic obstruction
  - Calcium channel blockers may also be useful in certain patients
  - For those who fail drug therapy, myectomy or dual-chamber pacing should be considered
  - The natural history of HOCM is unpredictable

Restrictive Cardiomyopathy

■ **Essentials of Diagnosis**

- This group of disorders is characterized by impaired diastolic filling with preserved left ventricular function
- The most common diseases in this category include amyloidosis, sarcoidosis, hemochromatosis, scleroderma, carcinoid syndrome, endomyocardial fibrosis, and postradiation fibrosis
- Clinical manifestations are those of the underlying disorder and congestive heart failure, with right-sided symptoms and signs usually predominating
- Electrocardiography may show low voltage and nonspecific ST–T wave abnormalities
- Echocardiography shows increased wall thickness with preserved contractile function

■ **Differential Diagnosis**

- Constrictive pericarditis
If patients present with diastolic dysfunction:
- Hypertensive heart disease
- Hypertrophic obstructive cardiomyopathy
- Aortic stenosis
- Ischemic heart disease

■ **Treatment**

- Sodium restriction and diuretic therapy for patients with evidence of fluid overload
- Digitalis is not indicated unless systolic function becomes impaired or atrial fibrillation occurs
- Treat the underlying disease causing the restriction, if possible

1

Acute Rheumatic Fever

■ Essentials of Diagnosis

- A systemic immune process complicating group A beta-hemolytic streptococcal pharyngitis
- Usually affects children between the ages of 5 and 15 years
- Occurs 1–5 weeks after throat infection
- Diagnosis based on Jones criteria and confirmation of recent streptococcal infection
- Major Jones criteria: erythema marginatum, migratory polyarthritis, subcutaneous nodules, carditis, and Sydenham's chorea; the latter is the most specific, least sensitive
- Minor criteria: fever, arthralgias, rapid erythrocyte sedimentation rate, elevated C-reactive protein, and PR prolongation

■ Differential Diagnosis

- Rheumatoid arthritis
- Endocarditis
- Osteomyelitis
- Systemic lupus erythematosus
- Lyme disease
- Disseminated gonorrhea

■ Treatment

- Bed rest until vital signs and ECG become normal
- Salicylates reduce fever and joint complaints but do not affect the natural course of the disease
- If streptococcal infection is still present, penicillin is indicated
- Prevention of recurrent streptococcal pharyngitis in patients less than 25 years old

Cardiac Tamponade

■ Essentials of Diagnosis

- A life-threatening disorder that occurs when pericardial fluid accumulates under pressure; effusions that increase rapidly in size may cause an elevated intrapericardial pressure (> 15 mm Hg), leading to impaired cardiac filling and decreased cardiac output
- The most common causes include metastatic malignancy, uremia, viral or idiopathic pericarditis, and cardiac trauma
- Clinical manifestations include dyspnea, cough, tachycardia, hypotension, pulsus paradoxus, jugular venous distention, and distant heart sounds
- Electrocardiography usually shows low QRS voltage and occasionally electrical alternans; chest x-ray shows an enlarged cardiac silhouette with a "water-bottle" configuration if a large (> 250 mL) effusion is present
- Echocardiography is the initial study of choice and will clearly delineate the presence of an effusion; cardiac catheterization confirms the diagnosis if equalization of diastolic pressures in all four chambers occurs

■ Differential Diagnosis

- Tension pneumothorax
- Right ventricular infarction
- Severe left ventricular failure
- Constrictive pericarditis
- Restrictive cardiomyopathy

■ Treatment

- Immediate pericardiocentesis
- Volume expansion until pericardiocentesis is performed

Chronic Constrictive Pericarditis

- ### Essentials of Diagnosis
  - Chronic inflammation may cause a thickened fibrotic pericardium that impairs cardiac filling and decreases cardiac output
  - May follow tuberculosis, cardiac surgery, radiation therapy, or viral, uremic, or neoplastic pericarditis
  - Symptoms include gradual onset of dyspnea, fatigue, weakness, pedal edema, and abdominal swelling
  - Physical examination reveals tachycardia, elevated jugular venous distention with rapid y descent, Kussmaul's sign, hepatomegaly, ascites, "pericardial knock" following S_2, and peripheral edema
  - Chest x-ray reveals pericardial calcification in half of patients; electrocardiography may show low QRS voltage
  - Echocardiography can demonstrate a thick pericardium and normal left ventricular function; CT or MRI is more sensitive in revealing pericardial pathology

- ### Differential Diagnosis
  - Cardiac tamponade
  - Right ventricular failure (due to any cause)
  - Restrictive cardiomyopathy
  - Cirrhosis with ascites

- ### Treatment
  - Acute treatment usually includes gentle diuresis
  - Definitive therapy includes surgical stripping of the pericardium
  - Patients should be evaluated for tuberculosis

Cor Pulmonale

- **Essentials of Diagnosis**
  - Cor pulmonale is defined by right ventricular enlargement and eventual failure resulting from pulmonary disease
  - Most commonly due to COPD; other causes include pulmonary fibrosis, pneumoconioses, recurrent pulmonary emboli, primary pulmonary hypertension, sleep apnea, and kyphoscoliosis
  - Clinical manifestations are due to both the underlying pulmonary disease and the right ventricular failure
  - Chest x-ray reveals an enlarged right ventricle and pulmonary artery; electrocardiography may show right axis deviation and tall, peaked P waves (P pulmonale) in the face of low QRS voltage
  - Pulmonary function tests usually confirm the presence of underlying lung disease, and echocardiography will show right ventricular dilation but normal left ventricular function

- **Differential Diagnosis**

  Other causes of right ventricular failure:
  - Left ventricular failure (due to any cause)
  - Pulmonary stenosis
  - Left-to-right shunt causing Eisenmenger's syndrome

- **Treatment**
  - Treatment is directed at the pulmonary process causing the right heart failure
  - If frank right ventricular failure is present, treatment should include salt restriction, diuretics, and oxygen

Essential Hypertension

- ■ Essentials of Diagnosis
  - In most patients (95% of cases), no cause of hypertension can be found—this is termed "essential" hypertension
  - A chronic elevation in blood pressure (> 140/90 mm Hg) occurs in 15% of white adults and 30% of black adults in the United States
  - The pathogenesis is multifactorial: a combination of environmental, genetic, and neurohormonal factors are probably responsible
  - Most patients are asymptomatic; some, however, may complain of headache, epistaxis, or blurred vision if hypertension is severe
  - Most chemical and laboratory findings are referable to "target organ" damage: heart, kidney, brain, eyes, and peripheral arteries

- ■ Differential Diagnosis
  Secondary causes of hypertension:
  - Coarctation of the aorta
  - Renal insufficiency
  - Renal artery stenosis
  - Pheochromocytoma
  - Cushing's syndrome
  - Primary hyperaldosteronism
  - Chronic use of oral contraceptive pills

- ■ Treatment
  - The goal is to decrease blood pressure with a single agent (if possible) while minimizing side effects
  - Many experts recommend diuretics and beta-blockers as initial therapy, but considerable latitude is allowed for individual patients
  - Other agents that can be useful either alone or in combination include ACE inhibitors, calcium channel blockers, and alpha-blockers
  - If hypertension is refractory to medical treatment, evaluation for secondary causes should be considered

Deep Venous Thrombosis

- ■ Essentials of Diagnosis
    - Pain or tight feeling in the calf or thigh, occasionally associated with swelling
    - Up to half of patients may be asymptomatic in the early stages
    - Increased risk with congestive heart failure, recent surgery, neoplasia, oral contraceptive use, prolonged inactivity, obesity, or varicose veins
    - Physical signs unreliable
    - Doppler ultrasound and impedance plethysmography abnormal; venography is diagnostic
    - May be complicated by pulmonary thromboembolism

- ■ Differential Diagnosis
    - Calf strain or contusion
    - Cellulitis
    - Ruptured Baker cyst
    - Lymphatic obstruction

- ■ Treatment
    - Extremity elevation and bed rest
    - Anticoagulation with intravenous heparin (goal PTT twice normal) × 5 days followed by oral warfarin × 3–6 months
    - Subcutaneous low-molecular-weight heparin may be substituted for intravenous heparin
    - NSAIDs for associated pain and swelling

1

Atrial Myxoma

- ■ Essentials of Diagnosis
  - Usually originates in the intraventricular septum, with 80% growing into the left atrium
  - Fever, malaise, weight loss, dyspnea, acute vascular or neurologic deficit
  - Diastolic "tumor plop" or mitral stenosis-like murmur; signs of congestive heart failure and systemic embolization in many
  - Episodic pulmonary edema, classically when patient assumes an upright position
  - Leukocytosis, anemia, elevated erythrocyte sedimentation rate
  - MRI or echocardiogram demonstrates tumor

- ■ Differential Diagnosis
  - Subacute infective endocarditis
  - Lymphoma
  - Autoimmune disease
  - Mitral stenosis
  - Other causes of congestive heart failure

- ■ Treatment
  - Surgery usually curative

2

Pulmonary Diseases

Acute Respiratory Distress Syndrome (ARDS)

- Essentials of Diagnosis
  - ARDS is a physiologic and radiologic syndrome with an onset of 12–48 hours after severe systemic or pulmonary insult
  - Rapid onset of dyspnea and respiratory distress, commonly in setting of trauma, shock, or sepsis (one-third of ARDS patients initially present with sepsis syndrome)
  - Tachypnea, fever, crackles or rhonchi by auscultation (ie, $Pao_2/Fio_2 < 200$)
  - Arterial hypoxemia refractory to supplemental oxygen; hypercapnia and respiratory acidosis in impending respiratory failure
  - Diffuse alveolar and interstitial infiltrates by radiography, often sparing costophrenic angles
  - Normal pulmonary capillary wedge pressure
  - Most patients demonstrate evidence of multi-organ failure

- Differential Diagnosis
  - Cardiogenic pulmonary edema
  - Primary pneumonia of any cause
  - Bronchiolitis obliterans with organizing pneumonia (BOOP)

- Treatment
  - Treat underlying disease process (eg, antimicrobial drugs for sepsis)
  - Mechanical ventilation with supplemental oxygen; positive end-expiratory pressure usually required
  - Maintain low left ventricular filling pressure monitoring by Swan-Ganz catheter occasionally necessary
  - Supportive therapy including adequate nutrition and vigilance for other organ dysfunction
  - Mortality rate may be as high as 50%

Pleural Effusion

2

- ■ Essentials of Diagnosis
  - Pleuritic chest pain, dyspnea in some; may be asymptomatic
  - Decreased breath sounds, percussive dullness, and bronchial breathing above top of effusion
  - Layering of effusion on decubitus chest x-rays; thoracic ultrasonography occasionally required for confirmation

- ■ Differential Diagnosis
  - Atelectasis
  - Lobar consolidation
  - Chronic pleural thickening
  - Malignancy
  - Subdiaphragmatic process

- ■ Treatment
  - Diagnostic thoracentesis for evaluating cause, with pleural fluid glucose, protein, CBC, LDH, special stains and cultures necessary
  - Therapy guided by suspected cause
  - Pleural biopsy indicated in selected cases for diagnostic purposes (eg, tuberculosis, mesothelioma)

Spontaneous Pneumothorax

- ■ Essentials of Diagnosis
  - Abrupt onset of ipsilateral chest pain, sometimes referred to shoulder or arm, dyspnea
  - Hyperresonance and decreased breath sounds over involved hemithorax; tachycardia, hypotension and mediastinal shift toward contralateral side if tension pneumothorax is present
  - Chest x-ray diagnostic with retraction of lung from parietal pleura, often best seen by end-expiratory film when pneumothorax is small

- ■ Differential Diagnosis
  - Myocardial infarction
  - Pulmonary emboli
  - Pneumonia
  - Pericarditis

- ■ Treatment
  - Assessment for cause, eg, pneumocystis pneumonia, lung cancer, COPD
  - Immediate decompression by needle thoracostomy if tension is suspected
  - Spontaneous pneumothoraces of less than 15% followed by serial radiographs and observation for at least 2 days in the hospital; pneumothoraces greater than 15% should be assisted by aspiration of air through small catheter or by tube thoracostomy depending on clinical setting
  - Discontinue smoking
  - Risk of recurrence is 50%
  - Therapy for recurrent pneumothorax includes surgical pleurodesis or stapling of the ruptured blebs

Bronchiolitis Obliterans With Organizing Pneumonia (BOOP)

2

- **Essentials of Diagnosis**
  - Bronchiolitis obliterans occurs in various settings in adults: postinfectious (*Mycoplasma,* viral infection); after toxic fume inhalation; connective tissue associated; after organ transplantation; and idiopathic (ie, BOOP)
  - Usually characterized by an abrupt onset of symptoms including dry cough, dyspnea, flu-like prodrome with fever and weight loss
  - Dry crackles and wheezing by auscultation; clubbing rare
  - Restrictive function by pulmonary function study; hypoxemia
  - Chest radiograph typically shows patchy, bilateral alveolar infiltrates
  - Open or thoracoscopic lung biopsy necessary for precise diagnosis

- **Differential Diagnosis**
  - Idiopathic pulmonary fibrosis
  - AIDS-related lung infections
  - Congestive heart failure
  - Mycobacterial or fungal infection
  - Severe pneumonia due to bacteria, fungi, or tuberculosis

- **Treatment**
  - Corticosteroids effective in two-thirds of cases
  - Relapse common after short (< 6 months) steroid courses

Solitary Pulmonary Nodule

- ■ Essentials of Diagnosis
  - Twenty-five percent of cases of bronchogenic carcinoma present as a solitary pulmonary nodule; the 5-year survival rate detected in this form is 50%
  - Round or oval circumscribed lesion less than 5 cm in diameter surrounded by normal lung tissue
  - Central cavitation, calcification, or satellite lesions may be seen
  - Factors favoring benign lesion: age under 35 years, asymptomatic patient, size under 2 cm, presence of calcification, smooth margins by tomography, and satellite lesions
  - Factors suggesting malignancy: age over 45 years, presence of symptoms, size greater than 2 cm, lack of calcification, and indistinct margins
  - Skin tests, serologic studies, sputum cytologic examination rarely helpful
  - Comparison with old chest radiographs essential; follow-up with serial radiographs or CT scans often helpful, as may be CT density comparisons with known standards for malignancies

- ■ Differential Diagnosis
  - Benign causes: infectious granulomas, arteriovenous malformations, pseudotumors, fat pads, hamartomas
  - Malignant causes: primary lung malignancies, metastatic malignancy

- ■ Treatment
  - Resection of all lesions in persons over 35 years of age recommended unless calcification typical of benign lesion or documented radiographic stability for 2 years
  - Conservative observation ("watchful waiting") may be justified if benign lesions strongly suggested by clinical picture or if other contraindications for surgery present
  - Role of fine-needle aspiration uncertain because of false-negatives

Asthma

2

- ■ Essentials of Diagnosis
  - Episodic or chronic dyspnea or tightness in chest with wheezing, cough
  - Some patients manifest attacks triggered by inhalation of antigens (extrinsic)
  - Tachycardia, hyperpnea; prolonged expiratory time, wheezing, or distant breath sounds; if severe, pulsus paradoxus and cyanosis are present
  - Leukocytosis, eosinophilia common; mucus casts, eosinophils, and Charcot-Leyden crystals in sputum
  - Obstructive pattern by spirometry at least partially reversible with bronchodilators

- ■ Differential Diagnosis
  - Congestive heart failure
  - Chronic obstructive pulmonary disease
  - Pulmonary embolism
  - Foreign body aspiration
  - Pulmonary infection (eg, strongyloidiasis, aspergillosis)
  - Churg-Strauss syndrome
  - Anaphylaxis

- ■ Treatment
  - Acute treatment: supplemental oxygen, inhaled bronchodilators (β_2 agonists or anticholinergic agents), systemic corticosteroids, evaluation for precipitating cause
  - Subcutaneous epinephrine for severe cases in patients under 35 years of age; leukotriene antagonists may also be useful in selected cases, but precise role is yet to be determined
  - Chronic therapy: avoidance of known precipitants, regular use with inhaled bronchodilators or corticosteroids; systemic corticosteroids, oral theophylline, and inhaled cromolyn sodium in selected patients
  - Empiric oral antibiotics controversial

Chronic Obstructive Pulmonary Disease (COPD)

- ■ Essentials of Diagnosis
  - Acute or chronic dyspnea (emphysema) or chronic cough or sputum production (chronic bronchitis), nearly always in a heavy smoker; many patients have components of both
  - Hyperpnea, increased anteroposterior chest diameter, distant breath sounds, wheezes or rhonchi, cyanosis; clubbing relatively unusual
  - Hypoxemia and hypercapnia more pronounced with chronic bronchitis than emphysema
  - Hyperexpansion with decreased markings by chest radiography; variable findings of bullae, thin cardiac shadow
  - Airflow obstruction by spirometry; normal diffusing capacity (DLco) in bronchitis, reduced in emphysema

- ■ Differential Diagnosis
  - Asthma
  - Bronchiectasis
  - Congenital emphysema (α_1-antiprotease deficiency)
  - Cystic fibrosis

- ■ Treatment
  - Aggressive patient education (eg, discontinue cigarette use)
  - Clinical trial of inhaled bronchodilators
  - Pulmonary rehabilitation
  - Pneumococcal vaccination; yearly influenza vaccination
  - Supplemental oxygen for hypoxic patients
  - For acute exacerbations, treat as acute asthma and identify underlying precipitant; if patients have low baseline peak flow rates, antibiotics may be beneficial

Cystic Fibrosis

2

■ Essentials of Diagnosis

- A generalized autosomal recessive disorder of the exocrine glands, affecting one in 2500 Caucasians
- Cough, dyspnea, recurrent pulmonary infections often due to *Pseudomonas;* symptoms of malabsorption, infertility
- Increased thoracic diameter, distant breath sounds, rhonchi, clubbing, nasal polyps
- Hypoxemia; obstructive or mixed pattern by spirometry; decreased diffusing capacity
- Sweat chloride > 80 meq/L (> 60 meq/L if age < 20)

P aeruginosa

■ Differential Diagnosis

- Asthma
- Bronchiectasis
- Congenital emphysema (α_1-antiprotease deficiency)

■ Treatment

- Comprehensive multidisciplinary therapy required, including genetic and occupational counseling
- Inhaled bland aerosols and bronchodilators and chest physiotherapy
- Antibiotics for recurrent airway infections guided by cultures and sensitivities (high rate of resistant *Pseudomonas aeruginosa* and *Staphylococcus aureus* infections seen)
- Pneumococcal vaccination; yearly influenza vaccinations
- Recombinant human deoxyribonuclease given by aerosol is beneficial in many patients
- Lung transplantation is the definitive treatment in selected patients

Foreign Body Aspiration

- ■ Essentials of Diagnosis
  - Sudden onset of cough, wheeze, and dyspnea
  - Localized wheezing, hyperresonance and diminished breath sounds
  - Localized air trapping or atelectasis on end-expiratory chest radiography

- ■ Differential Diagnosis
  - Asthma with mucus plugging
  - Bronchiolitis
  - Pyogenic upper airway process (Ludwig's angina, soft tissue abscess, epiglottitis)
  - Laryngospasm associated with anaphylaxis
  - Bronchial compression from mass lesion
  - Substernal goiter

- ■ Treatment
  - Bronchoscopic or surgical removal of foreign body

Allergic Bronchopulmonary Aspergillosis

2

■ Essentials of Diagnosis

- Caused by an allergy to antigens of *Aspergillus* species that colonize the tracheobronchial tree
- Recurrent dyspnea, exacerbated by corticosteroid withdrawal, with history of asthma; cough productive of brownish plugs of sputum
- Physical examination as in asthma
- Peripheral eosinophilia, elevated serum IgE level, precipitating antibody to *Aspergillus* antigen present; positive skin hypersensitivity to *Aspergillus* antigen
- Infiltrate (often fleeting) and central bronchiectasis by chest radiography

■ Differential Diagnosis

- Asthma
- Bronchiectasis

■ Treatment

- Oral corticosteroids often required for several months
- Inhaled bronchodilators as for attacks of asthma
- Complications include hemoptysis, severe bronchiectasis, and pulmonary fibrosis

Bronchiectasis

- **Essentials of Diagnosis**
  - A congenital or acquired disorder affecting the large bronchi causing permanent abnormal dilation and destruction of bronchial walls
  - Chronic cough with copious purulent sputum, hemoptysis; weight loss, recurrent pneumonias
  - Coarse, moist crackles; clubbing
  - Hypoxemia with obstructive pattern by spirometry
  - Chest x-rays variable, may show multiple cystic lesions at bases in advanced cases
  - Thin-section CT scan helpful
  - Often associated with underlying systemic disorder (eg, cystic fibrosis, hypogammaglobulinemia), or chronic pulmonary infection (eg, tuberculosis, lung abscess)

- **Differential Diagnosis**
  - Chronic obstructive pulmonary disease
  - Tuberculosis
  - Chronic lung abscess
  - Pneumonia due to any cause

- **Treatment**
  - Discontinuation of smoking
  - Antibiotics selected by sputum culture and sensitivities
  - Chest physiotherapy
  - Inhaled bronchodilators
  - Surgical resection in selected patients with unresponsive localized disease or massive hemoptysis
  - Complications include cor pulmonale, amyloidosis, and secondary visceral abscesses (eg, brain abscess)

Acute Viral Bronchiolitis

2

- **Essentials of Diagnosis**
  - Rhinitis, cough, wheezing in children under 2 years age
  - Tachypnea, with intercostal retractions; wheezing
  - Pulmonary hyperaeration on chest x-ray
  - Respiratory syncytial virus is the most common cause

- **Differential Diagnosis**
  - Asthma
  - Inhalation of toxic fumes
  - Intrabronchial foreign body or tumor
  - Bacterial croup
  - Pertussis

- **Treatment**
  - Hospitalize patients who are under 2 months of age, have history of apnea, have $Po_2 < 60$ mm Hg, or have $Pco_2 > 45$ mm Hg
  - Inhaled bronchodilator therapy
  - Antibiotic therapy if suspected bacterial superinfection

Acute Tracheobronchitis

- ■ Essentials of Diagnosis
  - Poorly defined but common condition characterized by inflammation of the trachea and bronchi
  - Due to infectious agents (bacteria or viruses) or irritants (like dust and smoke)
  - Cough with pleuritic substernal chest pain
  - Symptoms of upper respiratory tract infection often precede the manifestations of tracheobronchitis
  - Variable rhonchi and wheezing; fever is usually absent
  - Chest x-ray normal
  - Increased incidence in smokers

- ■ Differential Diagnosis
  - Asthma
  - Pneumonia
  - Intrabronchial foreign body
  - Cystic fibrosis
  - Inhalation pneumonitis
  - Viral croup

- ■ Treatment
  - Symptomatic therapy with inhaled bronchodilators, cough suppressant
  - Antibiotics for purulent sputum directed by diagnostic Gram stain or sputum culture; empiric therapy for selected patients
  - Patients encouraged to stop smoking

Acute Bacterial Pneumonia

2

- **Essentials of Diagnosis**
  - Fever, chills, cough with purulent sputum production; early pleuritic pain, often severe, suggests pneumococcal etiology
  - Tachycardia, tachypnea; bronchial breath sounds with percussive dullness and egophony over involved lung; findings may be more pronounced after hydration
  - Leukocytosis with left shift
  - Patchy or lobar infiltrate by chest x-ray
  - Diagnostic Gram stain or culture of sputum, blood, or pleural fluid
  - Bacterial causes include *Streptococcus pneumoniae, Haemophilus influenzae,* gram-negative rods, *Staphylococcus aureus, Legionella*

- **Differential Diagnosis**   *S. pnewmo = rusty spatum*
  - Lung abscess
  - Pulmonary embolism
  - Myocardial infarction
  - Atypical pneumonia
  - Bronchiolitis obliterans with organizing pneumonia (BOOP)

- **Treatment**
  - Empiric antibiotics after obtaining cultures
  - Hospitalize selected patients (severe hypoxemia, more than one lobe involved, poor host resistance factors, presence of coexisting illness, leukopenia or marked leukocytosis, hypotension)
  - Pneumococcal vaccine can prevent or lesson the severity of pneumococcal infections in up to 90% of patients

Atypical Pneumonia

- ■ Essentials of Diagnosis
  - Cough with scant sputum, fever, malaise, headache; gastrointestinal symptoms variable
  - Nonspecific physical examination
  - Mild leukocytosis; cold agglutinins sometimes positive
  - Patchy, nonlobar infiltrate by chest x-ray often surprisingly extensive
  - Pathogens include *Mycoplasma, Chlamydia,* viral agents

- ■ Differential Diagnosis   ⌐ walking
                                pneumonia ⌐
  - Bacterial pneumonia
  - Pulmonary embolism
  - Congestive heart failure

- ■ Treatment
  - Empiric antibiotic treatment with erythromycin or tetracycline
  - Hospitalize as for bacterial pneumonia

Anaerobic Pneumonia & Lung Abscess

2

- ■ Essentials of Diagnosis
  - Cough producing foul-smelling sputum; hemoptysis; fever, weight loss, malaise
  - Patients with periodontal disease, history of impaired deglutition (eg, neurologic or esophageal disorder or altered consciousness) are predisposed
  - Bronchial breath sounds with dullness and egophony over involved lung; Hippocratic succussion splash in rare patients
  - Leukocytosis; hypoxia
  - Chest x-ray density often with central lucency or air-fluid level
  - Sputum cultures reveal only mouth flora

- ■ Differential Diagnosis
  - Tuberculosis
  - Bronchogenic carcinoma
  - Pulmonary mycoses
  - Bronchiectasis
  - Cavitary bacterial pneumonia
  - Pulmonary vasculitides (eg, Wegener's granulomatosis)
  - Foreign body

- ■ Treatment
  - Long-term clindamycin or high-dose penicillin
  - Postural drainage, inhaled bronchodilators
  - Surgery in selected cases (massive abscess; massive or persistent hemoptysis)
  - Supplemental oxygen as needed
  - Bronchoscopic exclusion of carcinoma or foreign body aspiration in patients with atypical features, especially edentulous patients

Pulmonary Tuberculosis

- ■ **Essentials of Diagnosis**
  - Lassitude, weight loss, fever, cough, night sweats, hemoptysis; may be asymptomatic, however
  - Patient may appear chronically ill and exhibit evidence of weight loss; posttussive apical rales occasionally present
  - Apical or subapical infiltrates with cavities classic in reactivation tuberculosis; pleural effusion in primary, but any radiographic abnormality is possible
  - Positive skin test to intradermal purified protein derivative (PPD) in majority of cases
  - *Mycobacterium tuberculosis* by culture of sputum, pleural fluid, gastric washing, or pleural biopsy
  - Granuloma on pleural biopsy for patients with effusions

- ■ **Differential Diagnosis**
  - Bronchogenic carcinoma
  - Pneumonia or lung abscess
  - Sarcoidosis
  - Pneumoconioses
  - Other mycobacterial infections in patients not immunosuppressed
  - Melioidosis

- ■ **Treatment**
  - Combination antituberculous therapy for 6–9 months; all regimens include isoniazid, but rifampin, ethambutol, pyrazinamide, streptomycin all have activity
  - All cases of suspected *M tuberculosis* infection reported to local health departments
  - Hospitalization should be considered for those incapable of self-care or likely to expose susceptible individuals

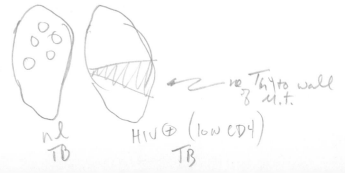

Idiopathic Pulmonary Fibrosis (Cryptogenic Fibrosing Alveolitis)

2

- ■ Essentials of Diagnosis
  - The most common disease among those presenting with interstitial lung disease
  - Insidious onset of dyspnea, dry cough in patients usually in their sixth or seventh decades
  - Paninspiratory crackles by auscultation; clubbing
  - Hypoxemia, especially exertional; antinuclear antibody and rheumatoid factor determinations frequently positive
  - Diffuse interstitial infiltration by chest x-ray which may progress to "honeycombing" pattern
  - Restrictive pattern by spirometry with decreased diffusing capacity (DLco)
  - Thin-section CT scan of the chest often helpful
  - Transbronchial or thoracoscopic lung biopsy shows patchy or diffuse alveolitis with fibrosis of alveolar septum
  - Diagnosis is based on clinical presentation after excluding other diagnoses

- ■ Differential Diagnosis
  - Bronchiolitis obliterans organizing pneumonia (BOOP)
  - Interstitial lung disease due to infection (eg, tuberculosis or fungus)
  - Drug-induced fibrosis (eg, secondary to bleomycin, nitrofurantoin)
  - Sarcoidosis
  - Pneumoconioses (Asbestosis, silicosis, etc...)

- ■ Treatment
  - Supportive therapy including supplemental oxygen
  - High-dose oral corticosteroids are usual therapy, particularly if active inflammation noted on biopsy and infection excluded
  - Cytotoxic therapy, lung transplantation reported successful in selected cases
  - Five-year survival is 50%

Sarcoidosis

- ■ Essentials of Diagnosis

  - A systemic disease of unknown cause with an increased incidence in North American blacks and North European whites
  - Malaise, fever, dyspnea of insidious onset; symptoms referable to eyes, skin, nervous system, liver, or heart also common; very often presents asymptomatically, however
  - Iritis, erythema nodosum, parotid enlargement, lymphadenopathy, hepatosplenomegaly; occasionally dry crackles by auscultation
  - Lymphopenia, eosinophilia, elevated erythrocyte sedimentation rate; hypercalcemia (5%) less common than hypercalciuria (20%)
  - Pulmonary function testing may show evidence of obstruction but restriction with decreased DLco is more commonly found
  - Symmetric hilar and right paratracheal adenopathy, interstitial infiltrates, or a combination of both seen on chest x-ray
  - Tissue reveals noncaseating granuloma; transbronchial biopsy gives highest yield, even without parenchymal disease on chest film
  - Increased angiotensin-converting enzyme levels are neither sensitive nor specific

- ■ Differential Diagnosis

  - Tuberculosis
  - Lymphoma
  - Histoplasmosis
  - Coccidioidomycosis
  - Idiopathic pulmonary fibrosis
  - Pneumoconioses
  - HIV disease
  - Berylliosis

- ■ Treatment

  - Oral systemic corticosteroid therapy for symptomatic pulmonary disease, cardiac involvement, iritis unresponsive to local therapy, arthritis, hypercalcemia, dermopathy, meningitis

Pulmonary Thromboembolism

2

- **Essentials of Diagnosis**
  - Abrupt onset of dyspnea and anxiety, pleuritic chest pain, cough with hemoptysis; syncope rare, but suggestive of extensive disease
  - Tachycardia, tachypnea, commonest findings; loud P_2 with right-sided S_3 characteristic but unusual; findings of peripheral venous thrombosis often absent
  - Acute respiratory alkalosis and hypoxemia
  - Characteristic perfusion defect on ventilation-perfusion scan, confirmed by pulmonary angiography in selected patients

- **Differential Diagnosis**
  - Pneumonia
  - Myocardial infarction
  - Atelectasis
  - Any cause of acute respiratory distress (eg, pneumothorax, aspiration, pulmonary edema, or asthma)

- **Treatment**
  - Anticoagulation: acutely with heparin, instituting warfarin concurrently for a minimum of 6 weeks
  - Thrombolytic therapy initially in selected patients with hemodynamic compromise
  - Intravenous filter placement in inferior vena cava for selected patients not candidates for or unresponsive to anticoagulation

Primary Pulmonary Hypertension

- ■ Essentials of Diagnosis
    - A rare disorder seen primarily in young and middle-aged women
    - Defined as pulmonary hypertension and elevated peripheral vascular resistance in the absence of other disease of the lung or heart
    - Progressive dyspnea, malaise, chest pain, exertional syncope
    - Tachycardia, increased P_2, systolic ejection click, right-sided S_3; may have evidence of right-sided failure (peripheral edema, hepatomegaly, ascites)
    - Right ventricular strain or hypertrophy by electrocardiography
    - Large central pulmonary arteries by chest x-ray
    - Must exclude treatable secondary causes of pulmonary hypertension like left ventricular failure, sleep apnea, pulmonary embolism

- ■ Differential Diagnosis
    - Mitral stenosis
    - Chronic pulmonary embolism
    - Collagen-vascular disease
    - Ischemic heart disease
    - Congenital heart disease
    - Cirrhosis of the liver

- ■ Treatment
    - Empiric anticoagulation may confer survival benefit
    - Vasodilator agents of unpredictable and uncertain efficacy
    - Heart-lung transplantation is an option since overall prognosis is very poor

Silicosis

2

- **Essentials of Diagnosis**
  - A typical pneumoconiosis, which is a chronic fibrotic lung disease caused by the inhalation of various dusts
  - History of extensive prolonged exposure to dust containing silicon dioxide (eg, foundry work, sandblasting, hard rock mining)
  - Progressive dyspnea, often over months to years
  - Dry inspiratory crackles by auscultation
  - Characteristic changes on chest radiograph with bilateral fibrosis and nodules (upper greater than lower lobes), and hilar lymphadenopathy with "eggshell" calcification
  - Pulmonary function studies yield mixed obstructive and restrictive pattern

- **Differential Diagnosis**
  - Other inhalation pneumoconioses (eg, asbestosis)
  - Tuberculosis (often complicates silicosis)
  - Sarcoidosis
  - Histoplasmosis
  - Coccidioidomycosis
  - Idiopathic pulmonary fibrosis

- **Treatment**
  - Supportive care only, with home oxygen if sustained hypoxemia present
  - Chemoprophylaxis with isoniazid necessary for all silicotic patients with positive tuberculin reactivity, given the increased incidence of tuberculosis

Asbestosis

- ■ Essentials of Diagnosis
  - History of exposure to dust containing asbestos particles (ie, mining, insulation, construction, shipbuilding)
  - Progressive dyspnea, rarely pleuritic chest pain
  - Dry inspiratory crackles common; clubbing and cyanosis occasionally seen
  - Interstitial fibrosis, later coalescing into nodules, is characteristic (lower field greater than upper field); pleural thickening, plaques, or diaphragmatic calcification common but unrelated to parenchymal disease; in some, exudative pleural effusion develops before parenchymal disease
  - Thin-section CT scan often confirmatory
  - Pulmonary function testing shows a restrictive defect with a diminished DLco often the earliest abnormality
  - Increased incidence of lung carcinoma and mesothelioma noted; cigarette smoking increases risk of former only

- ■ Differential Diagnosis
  - Other inhalation pneumoconioses (eg, silicosis)
  - Tuberculosis
  - Sarcoidosis
  - Histoplasmosis
  - Coccidioidomycosis
  - Idiopathic pulmonary fibrosis

- ■ Treatment
  - Supportive only, with oxygen supplementation for sustained hypoxemia

Pulmonary Alveolar Proteinosis

2

- ■ Essentials of Diagnosis
  - Progressive dyspnea and low-grade fever
  - Physical examination often normal
  - Hypoxemia, bilateral alveolar infiltrates suggestive of pulmonary edema on chest radiography
  - Characteristic intra-alveolar phospholipid accumulation without fibrosis at open lung biopsy
  - May be idiopathic or secondary (ie, post lung infection, immuno-compromised host)
  - Superinfection with *Nocardia* may be observed

- ■ Differential Diagnosis
  - Congestive heart failure
  - Acute pneumonia
  - Bronchiolitis obliterans with organizing pneumonia (BOOP)

- ■ Treatment
  - Periodic whole lung lavage reduces exertional dyspnea
  - Natural history variable, with occasional spontaneous remissions seen

Eosinophilic Pneumonia

■ Essentials of Diagnosis

- Fever, dry cough, wheezing, dyspnea, and weight loss variable from transient to severe and progressive
- Wheezing, dry crackles occasionally appreciated by auscultation
- Peripheral blood eosinophilia present in most cases
- Peripheral pulmonary infiltrates by radiograph in many cases (ie "the radiologic negative" of pulmonary edema) shown to be eosinophilic by bronchoalveolar lavage or open lung biopsy
- Some cases associated with L-tryptophan

■ Differential Diagnosis

- Acute infectious pneumonia
- Asthma
- Idiopathic pulmonary fibrosis
- Bronchiolitis obliterans with organizing pneumonia (BOOP)
- Churg–Strauss syndrome

■ Treatment

- Removal of offending drug
- Corticosteroid therapy often yields dramatic positive results in idiopathic cases; recurrence is common

Sleep-Related Breathing Disorders

2

- **Essentials of Diagnosis**
  - Excessive daytime somnolence or fatigue, morning headache, weight gain, impotence; bed partner may report restless sleep and loud snoring
  - Obesity, systemic hypertension common; signs of pulmonary hypertension or cor pulmonale develop over time
  - Erythrocytosis common
  - Sleep studies show periods of apnea, and bradycardia often marked
  - Most cases are of mixed central or obstructive origin; pure central sleep apnea is rare

- **Differential Diagnosis**
  - Alcohol or sedative abuse
  - Narcolepsy
  - Depression
  - Seizure disorder
  - Chronic obstructive pulmonary disease
  - Hypothyroidism

- **Treatment**
  - Weight loss and avoidance of sedatives or hypnotic medications mandatory
  - Nocturnal nasal continuous positive airway pressure (CPAP) and supplemental oxygen frequently abolish obstructive apnea
  - Protriptyline or medroxyprogesterone acetate effective in some of patients
  - Surgical approaches (uvulopalatopharyngoplasty, nasal septoplasty, tracheostomy) reserved for selected severe or refractory cases

3

Gastrointestinal Diseases

Gastroesophageal Reflux Disease (Reflux Esophagitis)

- **Essentials of Diagnosis**
  - Substernal burning (pyrosis) or pressure, aggravated by recumbency and relieved with sitting; waterbrash, dysphagia; nocturnal regurgitation, cough, or wheezing common
  - Esophageal reflux or hiatal hernia may be found by fluoroscopy at barium study; iron deficiency anemia secondary to occult blood loss may be encountered
  - Manometry reveals incompetent lower esophageal sphincter; endoscopy with biopsy may be necessary for diagnosis
  - Esophageal pH monitoring and acid perfusion (Bernstein) tests sometimes helpful
  - Conditions associated with diminished lower esophageal sphincter tone include obesity, pregnancy, hiatal hernia, nasogastric tube, recurrent emesis, Raynaud's phenomenon, and use of calcium channel antagonists

- **Differential Diagnosis**
  - Peptic ulcer disease
  - Cholecystitis
  - Angina pectoris
  - Achalasia
  - Esophageal spasm
  - Myocardial infarction
  - Pericarditis

- **Treatment**
  - Weight loss if indicated, avoidance of late night meals, elevation of head of bed
  - Avoid substances reducing lower esophageal sphincter tone (chocolate, caffeine, tobacco, alcohol, fried or fatty foods)
  - Antacids, high-dose H_2 antagonists, or proton pump inhibitors (eg, omeprazole)
  - Gastrointestinal motility stimulants (eg, bethanechol, metoclopramide, cisapride) in selected patients
  - Operative repair via abdominal (Hill, Nissen) or thoracic (Belsey) approach for rare cases refractory to medical management

Esophageal Aperistalsis

3

- ■ Essentials of Diagnosis
    - Dysphagia, substernal fullness or burning (pyrosis)
    - Absence of esophageal motor activity by fluoroscopic or manometric studies
    - Associations include Raynaud's phenomenon, scleroderma, SLE, polymyositis, or advanced age

- ■ Differential Diagnosis
    - Angina pectoris
    - Achalasia
    - Benign lower esophageal stricture
    - Diffuse esophageal spasm
    - Esophageal or mediastinal tumor

- ■ Treatment
    - Management as for reflux esophagitis

Diffuse Esophageal Spasm

- ■ Essentials of Diagnosis
  - Dysphagia, substernal pain, hypersalivation, reflux of recently ingested food
  - May be precipitated by ingestion of hot or cold foods
  - Endoscopic, radiographic, and manometric demonstration of non-propulsive hyperperistalsis; lower esophageal sphincter relaxes normally
  - "Nutcracker esophagus" variant with prolonged, high pressure (> 175 mm of mercury) propulsive contractions

- ■ Differential Diagnosis
  - Angina pectoris
  - Esophageal or mediastinal tumors
  - Aperistalsis
  - Achalasia
  - Psychoneurosis

- ■ Treatment
  - Nitrates often effective
  - Esophageal myotomy for refractory patients with severe disease

Achalasia

3

- ■ Essentials of Diagnosis
  - Progressive dysphagia, odynophagia, and regurgitation of undigested food
  - Barium swallow demonstrates a dilated upper esophagus with a narrowed cardioesophageal junction ("bird's beak" esophagus); chest x-ray may reveal a retrocardiac air-fluid level
  - Absent primary peristalsis by manometry or cineradiography and incomplete lower esophageal sphincter relaxation with swallowing

- ■ Differential Diagnosis
  - Diffuse esophageal spasm
  - Aperistalsis
  - Benign lower esophageal stricture
  - Esophageal or mediastinal tumors (esophageal carcinoma may complicate achalasia, however)
  - Scleroderma esophagus

- ■ Treatment
  - Nifedipine, 10–20 mg sublingually 30 minutes before meals
  - Pneumatic esophageal dilation
  - Surgical extramucosal myotomy (esophagocardiomyotomy) in refractory cases
  - Consider yearly esophagoscopy to evaluate for carcinoma

Cricopharyngeal Achalasia

- ■ Essentials of Diagnosis
  - Fullness felt in upper throat, regurgitation of recently ingested food
  - Cricopharyngeal bar on barium swallow
  - Upper esophageal sphincter dysfunction by manometry

- ■ Differential Diagnosis
  - Incompetence or stricture of lower esophageal sphincter
  - Esophageal or mediastinal tumor
  - Zenker's diverticulum (occasionally associated)
  - Achalasia
  - Aperistalsis

- ■ Treatment
  - Exclude lower esophageal sphincter dysfunction
  - Cricopharyngeal and upper esophageal myotomy for patients with hypertonic upper esophageal sphincter

Epiphrenic Esophageal Diverticulum

■ Essentials of Diagnosis

- Dysphagia, sensation of pressure in lower esophagus after eating with intermittent vomiting
- Typical radiologic contour by barium study; disturbed motility of lower esophagus by manometry
- Occasionally associated hiatal hernia

■ Differential Diagnosis

- Achalasia
- Esophageal spasm
- Esophageal web
- Esophageal or mediastinal tumor

■ Treatment

- Surgical resection for severe symptoms
- Concomitant esophageal myotomy if motor disorder associated

Traction Esophageal Diverticulum

- ■ Essentials of Diagnosis
  - Usually incidental radiographic finding without symptoms
  - Rarely, dysphagia with episodic coughing caused by fixation of diverticulum to mediastinal structures
  - Barium study shows one or more diverticula

- ■ Differential Diagnosis
  - Esophageal or mediastinal tumor
  - Benign esophageal stricture

- ■ Treatment
  - None in most cases
  - Surgical excision if severely symptomatic
  - If suspected, endoscopy should be performed cautiously to avoid entering and perforating diverticulum

Esophageal Web

- ■ Essentials of Diagnosis
    - • Dysphagia
    - • Barium swallow (lateral view often required), esophagoscopy diagnostic
    - • Plummer-Vinson syndrome if associated with iron deficiency anemia, glossitis, and spooning of nails; may be higher incidence of hypopharyngeal carcinoma

- ■ Differential Diagnosis
    - • Achalasia
    - • Esophageal diverticulum
    - • Aperistalsis
    - • Esophageal or mediastinal tumor
    - • Esophageal stricture

- ■ Treatment
    - • Esophagoscopy with disruption of webs adequate in most cases
    - • Bougienage required on occasion

Benign Stricture of Esophagus

- ■ Essentials of Diagnosis
  - Dysphagia, odynophagia
  - Smooth narrowing of lumen radiographically; esophagoscopy and biopsy or cytology mandatory to exclude malignancy
  - Onset months to years following esophageal insult, eg, peptic esophagitis, indwelling nasogastric tube, corrosive ingestion, infectious esophagitis, or endoscopic injury

- ■ Differential Diagnosis
  - Achalasia
  - Esophageal or mediastinal tumor
  - Esophageal web
  - Schatzki's ring

- ■ Treatment
  - Monthly bougienage dilation definitive therapy for most patients
  - Surgical therapy required rarely

Barrett's Esophagus

■ Essentials of Diagnosis

- Occurs in up to 10% of patients with reflux esophagitis
- Dysphagia, heartburn, regurgitation
- Upper endoscopy with biopsy reveals columnar epithelium replacing squamous epithelium
- May be complicated by esophageal stricture or, in area of columnar epithelium, ulceration
- Esophageal adenocarcinoma may develop in up to 10% of patients

■ Differential Diagnosis

- Achalasia
- Esophageal or mediastinal tumor
- Esophageal web

■ Treatment

- Antacids, H_2 antagonists or omeprazole
- Surgical fundoplication in selected patients
- Surveillance esophagoscopy with biopsy at 1–2 year intervals

Corrosive Esophagitis

- ■ Essentials of Diagnosis
  - History of ingestion of caustic liquid or solid
  - Oral, pharyngeal, or substernal pain; odynophagia
  - Burns of lips, mouth, and tongue; drooling in severe cases

- ■ Differential Diagnosis
  - Rarely misdiagnosed

- ■ Treatment
  - Supportive care with fluids, analgesics, prevention of emesis
  - Acute use of esophagoscopy, antibiotics, and steroids is controversial
  - Surveillance for and management of late stricture development
  - Esophagogastrectomy with colonic interposition for severe injuries is required acutely on rare occasions

Mallory-Weiss Syndrome (Mucosal Laceration of the Gastroesophageal Junction)

3

- ■ Essentials of Diagnosis
  - Hematemesis of bright red blood, often following prolonged or forceful vomiting or retching
  - Common in alcoholics, pregnancy; bleeding in latter usually trivial because of low portal pressures
  - Endoscopic demonstration of vertical mucosal tear at cardioesophageal junction or proximal stomach
  - Hiatal hernia often concomitant

- ■ Differential Diagnosis
  - Peptic ulcer with hemorrhage
  - Esophageal varices
  - Gastritis with hemorrhage

- ■ Treatment
  - Usually none required, with spontaneous resolution of bleeding, unless concomitant varices present
  - Endoscopic hemostatic intervention or, rarely, surgery required for uncontrolled bleeding

Instrumental Perforation of the Esophagus

- ■ Essentials of Diagnosis
  - History of recent instrumentation (esophagogastroduodenoscopy, sclerotherapy) with sudden onset of pain in neck, chest, or abdomen and dyspnea; change in voice to lower pitch
  - Fever, systemic toxicity, subcutaneous emphysema, mediastinal crunch
  - Chest x-ray may reveal mediastinal air or pneumothorax
  - Elevated amylase of salivary origin—from saliva entering mediastinum through perforation
  - Localization of injury by fluoroscopic study with water-soluble opaque media

- ■ Differential Diagnosis
  - Mediastinal tumor, if chronic abscess complicates small perforation; otherwise, seldom a difficult diagnosis

- ■ Treatment
  - Immediate surgical closure, if possible
  - External drainage
  - Antibiotics to cover mouth flora

Emetogenic Esophageal Perforation (Boerhaave's Syndrome)

3

- ■ Essentials of Diagnosis
  - Often history of alcoholic binge drinking, excessive food intake, or both
  - Violent vomiting or retching followed by sudden pain in chest or abdomen
  - Fever, shock, subcutaneous emphysema, mediastinal crunch, rigid abdomen
  - Chest x-ray often reveals mediastinal widening or emphysema, pneumothorax; hyperamylasemia
  - Demonstration of rupture of lower esophagus by esophagogram with water-soluble opaque media

- ■ Differential Diagnosis
  - Myocardial infarction
  - Pulmonary embolism
  - Aortic dissection
  - Ruptured viscus
  - Acute pancreatitis
  - Shock due to other causes

- ■ Treatment
  - Aggressive supportive measures and broad-spectrum antibiotics covering mouth organisms
  - Thoracotomy with repair if diagnosis established within 24 hours
  - After 24 hours, surgical resection of site of perforation with creation of a temporary cervical esophagostomy and ligation of the cardia with feeding jejunostomy, followed later by colonic interposition

Foreign Bodies in the Esophagus

- **Essentials of Diagnosis**
  - Recent ingestion of food or foreign material
  - Vague discomfort in chest or neck, dysphagia, inability to handle secretions
  - Radiographic or endoscopic evidence of esophageal obstruction by foreign body

- **Differential Diagnosis**
  - Esophageal stricture
  - Esophageal or mediastinal tumor
  - Angina pectoris

- **Treatment**
  - Endoscopic removal

Periesophageal Hiatal Hernia

3

- ■ Essentials of Diagnosis
    - Esophagogastric junction and a portion of the gastric fundus protrudes through a hiatus in the crural diaphragm into the chest
    - Often asymptomatic or associated with gastroesophageal reflux disease, dyspepsia, and decreased pressure of the lower esophageal sphincter
    - May be complicated by dysphagia, gastric incarceration, stasis, or gastric ulcer
    - Radiographic studies diagnostic

- ■ Differential Diagnosis
    - Gastric or esophageal malignancy
    - Peptic ulcer disease
    - Ischemic heart disease

- ■ Treatment
    - Laparoscopic repair with anterior gastropexy (herniated stomach is sutured to posterior rectus sheath) for symptomatic patients

Gastritis

- ■ Essentials of Diagnosis
  - Symptoms often vague and include nausea, vomiting, anorexia, nondescript upper abdominal distress; significant hemorrhage may occur with or without other symptoms
  - Mild epigastric tenderness to palpation; in some, physical signs absent
  - Iron deficiency anemia on occasion
  - Endoscopy with gastric biopsy for definitive diagnosis
  - Multiple associations include stress (burns, sepsis, critical illness), drugs (NSAIDs, salicylates), atrophic states (aging, pernicious anemia), previous surgery (gastrectomy, Billroth II), *Helicobacter pylori* infection

- ■ Differential Diagnosis
  - Peptic ulcer
  - Hiatal hernia
  - Malignancy of stomach or pancreas
  - Cholecystitis
  - Ischemic cardiac disease

- ■ Treatment
  - Avoidance of alcohol, caffeine, salicylates, tobacco, and NSAIDs
  - Eradicate *Helicobacter pylori* if present
  - Antacids, H_2 receptor antagonists, proton pump inhibitors (in patients receiving oral feedings), or sucralfate
  - Prevention in high-risk patients (eg, patients in the intensive care unit with respiratory failure or a coagulopathy)

Duodenal Ulcer

■ **Essentials of Diagnosis**

- Epigastric pain 45–60 minutes following meals or nocturnal pain, both relieved by food or antacids, sometimes by vomiting; symptoms chronic and periodic; radiation to back common
- Iron deficiency anemia, positive fecal occult blood; amylase elevated with posterior penetration
- Ulcer crater or deformity of duodenal bulb demonstrated radiographically or endoscopically
- Caused by *Helicobacter pylori* in 90–95% of cases, NSAIDs in 5–10%, Zollinger-Ellison syndrome in less than 1%; *H pylori* infection may be diagnosed serologically
- Complications include hemorrhage, intractable pain, perforation, and obstruction

■ **Differential Diagnosis**

- Reflux esophagitis
- Gastritis
- Pancreatitis
- Cholecystitis
- Other peptic disease, ie, Zollinger-Ellison syndrome or gastric ulcer
- Ischemic cardiac disease

■ **Treatment**

- Eradicate *H pylori,* various multidrug regimens available
- Avoid tobacco, alcohol, xanthines, and ulcerogenic drugs, especially NSAIDs
- Antacids, H_2 receptor antagonists, proton pump inhibitors, or sucralfate
- Surgery may be needed for ulcers refractory to medical management (rare) or for the management of complications (eg, perforation, uncontrolled bleeding); supraselective vagotomy preferred unless patient unstable or is obstructed

Zollinger-Ellison Syndrome (Gastrinoma)

■ **Essentials of Diagnosis**

- Symptoms are those of severe, recurrent, intractable peptic ulcer disease
- Gastric acid hypersecretion; serum gastrin elevated to > 150 pg/mL (often much higher); abnormal secretin stimulation test
- Hyperchlorhydria, diarrhea common; latter relieved by nasogastric tubes
- Gastrinomas may arise in the pancreas, duodenum, or lymph nodes; over 50% are malignant but not usually aggressive
- Imaging studies may reveal ulcer in unusual site (distal duodenum or jejunum), though typical locations are more often affected
- May be associated with hyperparathyroidism and multiple endocrine neoplasia (MEN I)

■ **Differential Diagnosis**

- Peptic ulcer disease of other cause
- Esophagitis
- Gastritis
- Pancreatitis
- Cholecystitis
- Diarrhea or malabsorption from other causes

■ **Treatment**

- High-dose omeprazole
- Exploratory laparotomy for patients without preoperative evidence of unresectable metastatic disease
- Resection for localized disease
- Family counseling

3

Gastric Ulcer

- ■ Essentials of Diagnosis
  - Epigastric pain, unpredictably relieved by food or antacids; weight loss, anorexia, vomiting
  - Iron deficiency anemia, fecal occult blood positive
  - Ulcer demonstrated by barium study or endoscopy
  - Caused by *Helicobacter pylori* (in the majority of cases), NSAIDs, gastric malignancy, Zollinger-Ellison syndrome
  - Endoscopic biopsy or documentation of complete healing necessary to exclude gastric malignancy
  - Complications include hemorrhage, perforation, and obstruction

- ■ Differential Diagnosis
  - Other peptic ulcer disease
  - Gastric carcinoma
  - Cholecystitis
  - Esophagitis
  - Gastritis
  - Irritable or functional bowel disease
  - Ischemic cardiac disease

- ■ Treatment
  - Eradicate *H pylori* when present; various multidrug regimens available
  - Avoid tobacco, alcohol, xanthines, and ulcerogenic drugs, especially NSAIDs
  - Antacids, H_2 receptor antagonists, proton pump inhibitors, or sucralfate
  - Surgery may be needed for ulcers refractory to medical management (rare) or for the management of complications (eg, perforation, uncontrolled bleeding)

Stomal (Marginal) Ulcer

- ■ Essentials of Diagnosis
    - Symptoms of peptic ulcer disease in patient with history of previous operation for ulcer disease; pain often low or left-sided
    - Low epigastric tenderness with guarding; occasionally inflammatory mass palpable
    - Iron deficiency anemia, positive fecal occult blood
    - Endoscopy superior to radiography for visualization and diagnosis; most ulcers jejunal in location
    - Complications include hemorrhage, perforation, obstruction, and gastrojejunocolic fistula

- ■ Differential Diagnosis
    - Irritable bowel syndrome
    - Gastritis
    - Biliary disease
    - Pancreatitis
    - Recurrent peptic disease

- ■ Treatment
    - H_2 receptor antagonists or proton pump inhibitors
    - Operative treatment rarely necessary

Crohn's Disease

■ **Essentials of Diagnosis**

- Insidious onset, with intermittent bouts of diarrhea, low-grade fever, right lower quadrant pain; peripheral arthritis, spondylitis, rash less common but may be presenting symptoms
- Anemia, leukocytosis, positive fecal occult blood
- Complications include fistula formation, perianal disease with abscess, right lower quadrant mass and tenderness
- Radiographic findings of thickened, stenotic bowel with ulceration, stricturing, or fistulas; characteristic skip areas
- Histologic demonstration of submucosal inflammation with fibrosis and granulomatous lesions

■ **Differential Diagnosis**

- Ulcerative colitis
- Whipple's disease
- Appendicitis
- Diverticulitis
- Intestinal tuberculosis
- Mesenteric adenitis
- Lymphoma, other tumors of small intestine
- Miscellaneous arthropathies and skin diseases
- Infectious colitis

■ **Treatment**

- Low-residue, lactose-free diet, antidiarrheals, antispasmodics, vitamin B_{12} and calcium supplementation as needed
- Sulfasalazine for colonic disease
- Corticosteroids or mercaptopurine for acute flares or extraintestinal complications
- Surgery for refractory obstruction, fistula, or abscess

Celiac & Tropical Sprue

- ### Essentials of Diagnosis
  - Bulky, pale, frothy, greasy stools (steatorrhea); abdominal distention, flatulence, weight loss, and evidence of fat-soluble vitamin deficiencies
  - Hypochromic or megaloblastic anemia; abnormal D-xylose absorption; increased fecal fat
  - "Deficiency" pattern on small bowel radiographic studies; villous atrophy on small bowel biopsy

- ### Differential Diagnosis
  - Crohn's disease
  - Functional blind loop (especially jejunal diverticulosis)
  - Intestinal tuberculosis (may be associated with celiac sprue)
  - Intestinal lymphoma (may also complicate celiac sprue)
  - Whipple's disease
  - Pancreatic insufficiency

- ### Treatment
  - For tropical sprue: folic acid, vitamin B_{12} replacement if necessary, tetracycline or trimethoprim-sulfamethoxazole for 1–6 months
  - For celiac sprue: strict elimination of gluten from diet (ie, wheat, rye, barley, and oat products); vitamin supplementation (especially vitamin B_{12}) and steroids in selected patients

Disaccharidase (Lactase) Deficiency

- **Essentials of Diagnosis**
  - Symptoms vary from abdominal bloating, distention, cramps, and flatulence to explosive diarrhea in response to disaccharide ingestion
  - Stool pH < 5.5; reducing substances present in stool
  - Flat glucose response to disaccharide loading, abnormal hydrogen breath test, or resolution of symptoms on lactose-free diet suggests the diagnosis
  - Congenital in Asians and African–Americans; can also be secondary to acute enteritis of other causes

- **Differential Diagnosis**
  - Chronic mucosal malabsorptive disorders
  - Irritable bowel syndrome
  - Inflammatory bowel disease
  - Pancreatic insufficiency

- **Treatment**
  - Restriction of dietary lactose
  - Lactase enzyme (Lactaid) supplementation

Whipple's Disease

- **Essentials of Diagnosis**
  - Insidious onset of abdominal pain, malabsorption, lymphadenopathy, arthralgias, weight loss, steatorrhea, fever, polyarthritis, anemia, and mental status changes
  - Caused by infection with the bacillus *Tropheryma whippelii*
  - Small bowel mucosal biopsy reveals characteristic foamy mononuclear cells filled with periodic acid-Schiff staining (PAS) material; electron microscopy shows bacilli in multiple affected organs

- **Differential Diagnosis**
  - Celiac or tropical sprue
  - Crohn's disease
  - Ulcerative colitis
  - Intestinal lymphoma
  - Rheumatoid arthritis or B27 spondyloarthropathy

- **Treatment**
  - Antibiotic therapy with trimethoprim-sulfamethoxazole or ceftriaxone is first-line therapy
  - Treatment must be continued for at least 1 year

Intestinal Tuberculosis

■ **Essentials of Diagnosis**

- Chronic abdominal pain, anorexia, bloating; weight loss, fever, diarrhea, new-onset ascites in many
- Mild right lower quadrant tenderness; fistula-in-ano sometimes seen
- Barium study may reveal mucosal ulcerations or scarring and fibrosis with narrowing of the small or large intestine
- In peritonitis, fluid has high protein and mononuclear pleocytosis; peritoneal biopsy with granulomas, improvement if laparotomy performed
- Complications include intestinal obstruction, hemorrhage, fistula formation, and bacterial overgrowth with malabsorption

■ **Differential Diagnosis**

- Carcinoma of the colon or small bowel
- Inflammatory bowel disease
- Amebiasis (especially ameboma)
- Intestinal lymphoma
- Ovarian or peritoneal carcinomatosis
- *Mycobacterium avium-intracellulare* infection

■ **Treatment**

- Standard therapy for tuberculosis

Irritable Bowel Syndrome

■ Essentials of Diagnosis

- Chronic functional disorder characterized by abdominal pain, alteration in bowel habits, constipation and diarrhea often alternating, dyspepsia, anxiety or depression
- Variable abdominal tenderness
- Sigmoidoscopy may reveal spasm or mucous hypersecretion; other studies normal

■ Differential Diagnosis

- Inflammatory bowel disease
- Ischemic colitis
- Diverticular disease
- Peptic ulcer disease
- Pancreatitis

■ Treatment

- Reassurance and explanation
- High-fiber diet with or without fiber supplements; restricting dairy products may be helpful
- Antispasmodic agents (eg, dicyclomine, hyoscyamine, propantheline), antidiarrheal or anticonstipation agents
- Amitriptyline, behavioral modification with relaxation techniques helpful for some patients

Ulcerative Colitis

- **Essentials of Diagnosis**
  - Bloody diarrhea or diarrhea with mucus; tenesmus and cramping lower abdominal pain; associated with fever, weight loss, rash, peripheral arthritis, or spondylitis
  - Mild abdominal tenderness, mucocutaneous lesions, erythema nodosum; symptoms may improve with cigarette smoking
  - Anemia, leukocytosis, elevated sedimentation rate, hypoproteinemia, absent stool pathogens
  - Ragged mucosa with loss of haustral markings on barium enema; colon involved contiguously from rectum, rarely sparing it
  - Acute inflammatory changes with crypt abscesses on rectal mucosal biopsy
  - Increased incidence of adenocarcinoma in patients with long-standing active disease or pancolitis

- **Differential Diagnosis**
  - Bacterial or amebic colitis
  - Diverticular disease
  - Adenocarcinoma of the colon
  - Ischemic colitis
  - Pseudomembranous colitis
  - Granulomatous colitis

- **Treatment**
  - Topical mesalamine or corticosteroids by enema or suppository
  - Fiber supplements, lactose-free diet
  - Sulfasalazine, mesalamine, or olsalazine for chronic therapy
  - Mesalamine, corticosteroids, or cyclosporine for acute flares
  - Colectomy for toxic megacolon unresponsive to medical therapy, severe extracolonic manifestations, or, in selected patients, for cancer prophylaxis
  - Yearly follow-up with colonoscopy suggested

Polyps of the Colon & Rectum

- **Essentials of Diagnosis**
  - Discrete mass lesions arising from colonic epithelium and protruding into the intestinal lumen; polyps may be pedunculated or sessile
  - Most patients asymptomatic; can be associated with chronic occult blood loss
  - Family history may be present
  - Diagnosed by sigmoidoscopy, colonoscopy, or barium enema
  - Removing polyps decreases the incidence of adenocarcinoma

- **Differential Diagnosis**
  - Adenocarcinoma
  - Radiographic artifact

- **Treatment**
  - Surgical or endoscopic polypectomy in all cases with histologic review
  - Colectomy for familial polyposis or Gardner's syndrome
  - Surveillance colonoscopy every 3–5 years

Hemorrhoids

- **Essentials of Diagnosis**
  - Rectal bleeding, protrusion, pain
  - Mucoid discharge from rectum
  - Characteristic findings on external anal examination and anoscopy

- **Differential Diagnosis**
  - Rectal polyps
  - Carcinoma
  - Rectal prolapse

- **Treatment**
  - High-fiber diet, fiber supplements, stool softeners, Sitz baths, and anal suppositories
  - Hemorrhoidectomy for severe symptoms or complications
  - Injection therapy, rubber band ligation, or cryosurgery in selected patients

Anal Fissure (Fissura-in-Ano, Anal Ulcer)

- **Essentials of Diagnosis**
  - Linear disruption of the anal epithelium due to various causes
  - Rectal pain related to defecation; bleeding and constipation
  - Acute anal tenderness to digital examination
  - Ulceration and stenosis of anal canal, hypertrophic anal papilla, sentinel pile by anoscopy

- **Differential Diagnosis**
  - Rectal syphilis, tuberculosis, herpes, chlamydial infections
  - Crohn's disease
  - Malignant epithelioma or leukemia

- **Treatment**
  - High-fiber diet, psyllium, bran, stool softeners, Sitz baths, hydrocortisone suppositories
  - Local application of silver nitrate or gentian violet
  - Lateral internal sphincterotomy if no improvement with medical therapy

Acute Pancreatitis

- ### Essentials of Diagnosis
    - Abrupt onset of epigastric pain, often with radiation to the back; nausea, vomiting, fever, and dehydration
    - Abdominal tenderness, distention
    - History of previous episode, alcoholism, or biliary tract disease often present
    - Leukocytosis, elevated serum and urine amylase, hypocalcemia; hypertriglyceridemia (> 1000 mg/dL) may be causative, likewise hypercalcemia
    - Radiographic "sentinel loop" or "colon cutoff sign" may be seen on plain films of the abdomen

- ### Differential Diagnosis
    - Acute cholecystitis or cholangitis
    - Penetrating or perforating duodenal ulcer
    - Mesenteric infarction
    - Gastritis
    - Nephrolithiasis
    - Abdominal aortic aneurysm
    - Small bowel obstruction
    - Myocardial infarction

- ### Treatment
    - Withhold food and liquids by mouth
    - Nasogastric suction for severe pain, intravenous fluid and electrolyte replacement, analgesics, and antiemetics
    - Antibiotics for documented infection; discontinue drugs capable of causing the disease, eg, thiazides, corticosteroids
    - Aggressive surgical debridement for pancreatic necrosis
    - Endoscopic retrograde cholangiopancreatography with sphincterotomy for pancreatitis resulting from choledocholithiasis

Chronic Relapsing Pancreatitis

- ■ Essentials of Diagnosis
  - Persistent or recurrent abdominal pain
  - Pancreatic calcification by radiographic study
  - Pancreatic insufficiency with malabsorption and diabetes in a third of patients
  - Occurs in patients with alcoholism (most common), hereditary pancreatitis, or untreated hyperparathyroidism, or after abdominal trauma

- ■ Differential Diagnosis
  - Diabetes mellitus
  - Malabsorption due to other causes
  - Intractable duodenal ulcer
  - Carcinoma of the pancreas

- ■ Treatment
  - Low-fat diet, pancreatic enzyme supplements, avoidance of alcohol
  - Treatment of hyperlipidemia if present
  - Intravenous fluid and electrolyte replacement for acute exacerbations
  - Surgical therapy to restore free flow of bile or to treat intractable pain

4

Hepatobiliary Disorders

Viral Hepatitis

- **Essentials of Diagnosis**
  - Anorexia, nausea, vomiting, malaise, symptoms of flu-like syndrome, arthralgias, and aversion to smoking
  - Jaundice, fever; enlarged, tender liver
  - Normal to low white cell count; abnormal liver tests (ALT > AST) and liver function studies; serologic tests for hepatitis A (IgM antibody), hepatitis B (HBsAg), or hepatitis C may be positive
  - Liver biopsy shows characteristic hepatocellular necrosis and mononuclear infiltrates
  - Hepatitis A: oral transmission, short incubation period, good prognosis
  - Hepatitis B and hepatitis C: parenteral transmission, longer incubation period, progression to chronic disease more likely

- **Differential Diagnosis**
  - Alcoholic hepatitis
  - Leptospirosis
  - Secondary syphilis
  - Q fever
  - Choledocholithiasis
  - Carcinoma of the pancreas
  - Cholestatic jaundice secondary to drugs
  - Autoimmune hepatitis

- **Treatment**
  - Supportive care
  - Avoidance of hepatotoxins: alcohol, acetaminophen
  - Interferon-α for patients who develop symptomatic, chronic active hepatitis B or C

Autoimmune Hepatitis

- ■ Essentials of Diagnosis
    - Insidious onset; usually affects young women
    - Jaundice, spider nevi, hepatomegaly, acne, hirsutism, amenorrhea, abnormal liver function tests, increased aminotransferases, polyclonal gammopathy
    - Associated with arthritis, thyroiditis, nephritis, Coombs-positive hemolytic anemia
    - ANA or anti-smooth muscle antibody positive
    - Patients may develop cirrhosis

- ■ Differential Diagnosis
    - Chronic viral hepatitis
    - Sclerosing cholangitis
    - Primary biliary cirrhosis
    - Wilson's disease
    - Choledocholithiasis

- ■ Treatment
    - General supportive measures
    - Prednisone with or without azathioprine

Alcoholic Hepatitis

- **Essentials of Diagnosis**
  - Onset usually after years of alcohol intake; anorexia, nausea, abdominal pain
  - Jaundice, fever, hepatomegaly, ascites, encephalopathy
  - Macrocytic anemia, leukocytosis with left shift, thrombocytopenia, abnormal liver function tests (AST > ALT, increased bilirubin, prolonged prothrombin time), elevated serum gamma globulin level; AST rarely exceeds 300 IU/L despite severity of illness
  - Liver biopsy confirms diagnosis

- **Differential Diagnosis**
  - Cholecystitis, cholelithiasis
  - Cirrhosis
  - Fatty liver
  - Viral hepatitis

- **Treatment**
  - General supportive measures, withdrawal of alcohol, avoid hepatotoxins (acetaminophen)
  - Corticosteroids may be beneficial in severe disease when discriminant function (4.6 [Prothrombin time (PT) – control] + bilirubin [mg/dL]) is > 32

Cirrhosis

■ **Essentials of Diagnosis**

- Late, insidious onset of malaise, weight loss, abdominal pain or increasing abdominal girth, pruritus, impotence
- Jaundice, spider nevi, in some cases palpable firm hepatomegaly, palmar erythema, gynecomastia, ascites, edema, purpura, asterixis or encephalopathy
- Macrocytic anemia, thrombocytopenia, abnormal liver function studies (Prothrombin time (PT), albumin), abnormal liver tests, increased serum globulins
- Biopsy diagnostic with micro- or macronodular fibrosis
- Complications include varices, gastrointestinal bleeding, sepsis, encephalopathy, renal failure

■ **Differential Diagnosis**

- Hemochromatosis
- Primary biliary cirrhosis
- Congestive heart failure
- Constrictive pericarditis
- Wilson's disease

■ **Treatment**

- Supportive care, abstinence from alcohol, vitamin supplementation
- Diuretics or large-volume paracenteses for ascites and edema
- Antibiotic treatment and, debatably, prophylaxis for spontaneous bacterial peritonitis
- Lactulose for encephalopathy
- Transjugular intrahepatic portosystemic shunt for bleeding esophageal varices or refractory ascites
- Liver transplantation in selected cases

Primary Biliary Cirrhosis

■ Essentials of Diagnosis

- Usually affects women aged 40–60 with the insidious onset of pruritus, jaundice, and hepatomegaly
- Increased alkaline phosphatase, cholesterol, bilirubin; positive antimitochondrial antibody
- Complications include, steatorrhea, xanthomatous neuropathy, osteomalacia, osteoporosis, and portal hypertension

■ Differential Diagnosis

- Chronic biliary tract obstruction, ie, cholelithiasis-related stricture
- Bile duct carcinoma
- Inflammatory bowel disease complicated with cholestatic liver disease
- Sarcoidosis
- Alcohol-related cirrhosis
- Hemochromatosis

■ Treatment

- Cholestyramine, colestipol, or rifampin for pruritus
- Calcium and supplementation with vitamins A, K, and D
- Ursodeoxycholic acid, colchicine, or methotrexate may be helpful
- Liver transplant for refractory cirrhosis

Hemochromatosis

- ■ Essentials of Diagnosis
  - Autosomal recessive disease with symptoms of hepatic, pancreatic, and cardiac insufficiency; hypogonadism
  - Symptoms typically occur after age 50 in males and after age 60 in females with characteristic skin pigmentation, diabetes, and hepatomegaly
  - Hyperabsorption of iron and its parenchymal storage is causative
  - Elevated serum iron, transferrin, percentage saturation of iron, and ferritin; glucose intolerance; mildly abnormal AST and alkaline phosphatase
  - Liver biopsy characteristic, with positive iron stain identifying accumulation in parenchymal cells
  - Complications include cirrhosis, congestive heart failure, diabetes, impotence, arthropathy, hypopituitarism, and hepatocellular carcinoma

- ■ Differential Diagnosis
  - Other causes of cirrhosis
  - Other causes of congestive heart failure
  - Diabetes mellitus
  - Other causes of hypopituitarism

- ■ Treatment
  - Early recognition and diagnosis (precirrhotic state) is crucial
  - Weekly phlebotomy to deplete iron stores, followed by maintenance phlebotomy or intramuscular deferoxamine, an iron chelating agent
  - Treat complications of liver disease, congestive heart failure, diabetes, and arthropathy

Wilson's Disease (Hepatolenticular Degeneration)

- ■ Essentials of Diagnosis
  - Autosomal recessive disorder with onset between first and third decades and symptoms of acute or chronic liver or neuropsychiatric dysfunction
  - Excessive deposition of copper in the liver and brain
  - Kayser-Fleischer rings in the cornea, jaundice, hepatomegaly, parkinsonian tremor and rigidity, psychiatric abnormalities
  - Elevated urinary copper excretion (> 100 mg/24 h), elevated hepatic copper (> 100 mg/g), decreased serum ceruloplasmin (< 20 mg/dL); early in disease, low alkaline phosphatase

- ■ Differential Diagnosis
  - Other causes of hepatitis
  - Other causes of cirrhosis
  - Other causes of psychiatric and neurologic disturbances

- ■ Treatment
  - Restrict dietary copper (shellfish, organ foods, legumes)
  - Oral penicillamine facilitates urinary excretion of chelated copper
  - Trientine if penicillamine cannot be tolerated
  - Oral zinc acetate promotes fecal copper excretion
  - Pyridoxine supplement necessary with penicillamine treatment
  - Liver transplantation for fulminant hepatitis

Hepatic Vein Obstruction (Budd-Chiari Syndrome)

■ **Essentials of Diagnosis**
- Spectrum of disorders characterized by occlusion of the hepatic veins from a variety of causes
- Acute or chronic onset of tender, painful hepatic enlargement, jaundice, splenomegaly, and ascites
- Liver imaging studies may show a prominent caudate lobe, since its venous drainage may not be occluded; liver biopsy reveals characteristic central lobular congestion
- Venography demonstrates occlusion of the hepatic veins
- Associations include caval webs, polycythemia, right-sided heart failure, malignancy, "bush teas" (pyrrolizidine alkaloids), paroxysmal nocturnal hemoglobinuria, birth control pills, pregnancy

■ **Differential Diagnosis**
- Cirrhosis
- Constrictive pericarditis
- Restrictive cardiomyopathy

■ **Treatment**
- Treatment of complications, eg, ascites, encephalopathy
- Lifelong anticoagulation or treatment of underlying disease
- Mesocaval or mesoatrial shunt may be required
- Liver transplantation for severe hepatocellular dysfunction

4

Pyogenic Hepatic Abscess

4

- **Essentials of Diagnosis**
  - Right-sided or midabdominal pain, anorexia, nausea
  - Fever, jaundice, right upper quadrant tenderness
  - Leukocytosis with left shift; nonspecific abnormalities of liver function studies
  - Most common organisms are *Escherichia coli, Proteus vulgaris, Enterobacter aerogenes,* and anaerobic species
  - Elevated right hemidiaphragm by radiography; ultrasound, CT scan, or liver scan demonstrates intrahepatic defect

- **Differential Diagnosis**
  - Amebic hepatic abscess
  - Acute hepatitis
  - Right lower lobe pneumonia
  - Cholelithiasis, cholecystitis
  - Appendicitis

- **Treatment**
  - Antibiotics with coverage of gram-negative organisms and anaerobes
  - Needle or surgical drainage usually necessary

Amebic Hepatic Abscess

■ **Essentials of Diagnosis**

- Right-sided abdominal pain, right pleuritic chest pain; preceding or concurrent diarrheal illness in minority
- History of travel to endemic region
- Fever, tender palpable liver ("punch" tenderness), localized intercostal tenderness
- Anemia, leukocytosis with left shift, nonspecific liver test abnormalities
- Positive serologic tests for *Entamoeba histolytica* in over 95% of patients, though may be initially nondiagnostic
- Increased right hemidiaphragm by radiography; ultrasound, CT scan, or liver scan demonstrates location and number of abscesses

■ **Differential Diagnosis**

- Pyogenic abscess
- Acute hepatitis
- Right lower lobe pneumonia
- Cholelithiasis, cholecystitis
- Appendicitis

■ **Treatment**

- Metronidazole drug of choice; repeated courses occasionally necessary
- Percutaneous needle aspiration for toxic patient
- Oral course of iodoquinol following acute therapy to eradicate intestinal cyst phase

Cholelithiasis (Gallstones)

■ **Essentials of Diagnosis**

- Frequently asymptomatic but may be associated with recurrent bouts of right-sided or midepigastric pain and nausea or vomiting after eating
- Ultrasound, CT scan, and plain films demonstrate stones within the gallbladder
- Increased incidence with female gender, chronic hemolysis (sickle cell disease), obesity, Native American origin, inflammatory bowel disease, diabetes mellitus, pregnancy

■ **Differential Diagnosis**

- Acute cholecystitis
- Acute pancreatitis
- Peptic ulcer disease
- Acute appendicitis
- Acute hepatitis
- Right lower lobe pneumonia
- Myocardial infarction
- Radicular pain in T6–T10 dermatome

■ **Treatment**

- Laparoscopic or open cholecystectomy for symptomatic patients only
- Bile salts (cheno- and ursodeoxycholic acid) may cause dissolution of cholesterol stones
- Lithotripsy with concomitant bile salts may be successful

Choledocholithiasis

■ **Essentials of Diagnosis**

- Often a history of biliary tract disease; episodic attacks of right abdominal or epigastric pain that may radiate to the right scapula or shoulder; occasionally painless jaundice
- Pain, fever, and jaundice (Charcot's triad); associated with nausea, vomiting, hypothermia, shock, and leukocytosis with a left shift
- Elevated serum amylase and liver function tests, especially bilirubin and alkaline phosphatase
- Abdominal imaging studies may reveal gallstones
- Ultrasound or CT scan shows dilated biliary tree
- Endoscopic retrograde cholangiopancreatography (ERCP) localizes the degree and location of obstruction

■ **Differential Diagnosis**

- Carcinoma of the pancreas, ampulla of Vater, or common duct
- Acute hepatitis
- Biliary stricture
- Drug-induced cholestatic jaundice
- Pancreatitis
- Bacterial sepsis

■ **Treatment**

- Intravenous broad-spectrum antibiotics
- Endoscopic papillotomy and stone extraction followed by laparoscopic or open cholecystectomy
- A T tube may be placed in the common duct to decompress the common bile duct for at least 7–8 postoperative days

Biliary Stricture

- ■ Essentials of Diagnosis
  - Episodic cholangitis
  - Due to trauma from previous biliary tract surgery in 95% of cases
  - Transhepatic cholangiography or ERCP can demonstrate the stricture
  - Complications include acute cholangitis and secondary biliary cirrhosis

- ■ Differential Diagnosis
  - Choledocholithiasis
  - Drug-induced cholestasis
  - Carcinoma of pancreas or biliary tree
  - Hepatitis due to any cause

- ■ Treatment
  - Intravenous antibiotics for acute cholangitis
  - Surgical choledochojejunostomy or hepaticojejunostomy may be required to reestablish bile flow into the intestine
  - Stenting procedures can be used for patients at high risk for surgery

Sclerosing Cholangitis

- ### Essentials of Diagnosis
  - Progressively obstructive jaundice, pruritus, malaise, anorexia, and indigestion, most common in young men aged 20–40 years
  - Two-thirds of cases have associated ulcerative colitis
  - Positive antineutrophil cytoplasmic antibody found in 70%; elevated total bilirubin and alkaline phosphatase common
  - ERCP demonstrates thick or narrowed biliary ductal system
  - Absence of previous biliary stones, biliary surgery, congenital abnormalities, biliary cirrhosis, and cholangiocarcinoma necessary to make the diagnosis

- ### Differential Diagnosis
  - Choledocholithiasis
  - Drug-induced cholestasis
  - Carcinoma of pancreas or biliary tree
  - Hepatitis due to any cause

- ### Treatment
  - Corticosteroids and broad-spectrum antibiotics may be helpful
  - Ursodeoxycholic acid may improve liver function tests but does not alter natural history
  - Stenting or balloon dilation of localized strictures by ERCP
  - Liver transplantation for decompensated disease

5

Hematologic Diseases

Iron Deficiency Anemia

- ■ Essentials of Diagnosis
  - Lassitude; in children under age 2, poor muscle tone, delayed motor development
  - Pallor, cheilosis, and koilonychia
  - Hypochromic microcytic red cells
  - Serum iron low, total iron-binding capacity increased; absent marrow iron, serum ferritin less than 12 ng/mL
  - Occult blood loss invariably causative in adults

- ■ Differential Diagnosis
  - Anemia of chronic disease
  - Thalassemia
  - Sideroblastic anemia

- ■ Treatment
  - Oral ferrous sulfate or ferrous gluconate three times daily for 6–12 months
  - Parenteral iron dextran for selected patients with severe, clinically significant iron deficiency
  - Evaluation for occult blood loss

Anemia of Chronic Disease

- ■ Essentials of Diagnosis
    - Known chronic disease, particularly inflammatory; symptoms and signs usually those of responsible disease
    - Modest anemia (Hct ≥ 25%; red cells normal morphologically but may be slightly microcytic)
    - Low serum iron with normal or low total iron-binding capacity, normal or high serum ferritin, and normal or increased bone marrow iron stores

- ■ Differential Diagnosis
    - Iron deficiency anemia
    - Sideroblastic anemia
    - Thalassemia

- ■ Treatment
    - Treatment of the underlying disease
    - For severe cases, red blood cell transfusions, recombinant erythropoietin

Hypersplenism

- **Essentials of Diagnosis**
  - Splenomegaly
  - Pancytopenia; active bone marrow with normal cellular precursors and normal maturity

- **Differential Diagnosis**
  - Acute leukemia
  - Hodgkin's and non-Hodgkin's lymphomas
  - Aplastic anemia
  - Paroxysmal nocturnal hemoglobinuria
  - Cirrhosis
  - Disseminated infections and marrow infiltrative processes
  - AIDS

- **Treatment**
  - Splenectomy for pancytopenia due to splenic vein thrombosis or for recurrent infections or bleeding associated with leukopenia and thrombocytopenia
  - Pneumococcal vaccination presplenectomy

Agranulocytosis

- **Essentials of Diagnosis**
  - Chills, fever, sore throat, malaise of abrupt onset
  - Mucosal ulceration
  - History of drug ingestion (eg, propylthiouracil)
  - Granulocytopenia with relative lymphocytosis

- **Differential Diagnosis**
  - Aplastic anemia
  - Acute leukemia
  - Felty's syndrome

- **Treatment**
  - Discontinue all drugs
  - Broad-spectrum antibiotics for fever

5

Acute Hemolytic Anemia

- ■ Essentials of Diagnosis
  - Sudden onset with chills, fever, nausea, or pain in abdomen or back
  - Pallor, slight jaundice, splenomegaly on examination
  - Red or dark urine, increased serum indirect bilirubin, reticulocytosis, bite cells on peripheral smear
  - Causes include congenital enzyme deficiencies (eg, glucose 6 phosphate dehydrogenase, pyruvate kinase), autoimmune diseases (eg, systemic lupus erythematosus), neoplasm (eg, lymphoma), and infectious diseases (eg, clostridial sepsis, various viral illnesses, malaria)

- ■ Differential Diagnosis
  - Hereditary spherocytosis
  - Acquired autoimmune hemolytic anemia
  - Hemoglobinopathy
  - ABO incompatibility in newborns

- ■ Treatment
  - Transfusions for symptoms
  - Precipitating cause of hemolysis must be identified and treated
  - Splenectomy in some patients, particularly those with pyruvate kinase deficiency

Thalassemia Major

- ■ Essentials of Diagnosis
    - Severe anemia from infancy; positive family history
    - Massive hepatosplenomegaly
    - Hypochromic, microcytic red cells with severe poikilocytosis, target cells, acanthocytes, and basophilic stippling on smear
    - Greatly elevated hemoglobin F levels

- ■ Differential Diagnosis
    - Other hemoglobinopathies
    - Congenital nonspherocytic hemolytic anemia

- ■ Treatment
    - Regular red blood cell transfusions
    - Oral folic acid supplementation
    - Splenectomy for secondary hemolysis due to hypersplenism
    - Deferoxamine to avoid iron overload
    - Allogeneic bone marrow transplantation in selected cases

5

Beta-Thalassemia Minor

- ■ Essentials of Diagnosis
  - Symptoms variable depending on degree of anemia; no specific physical findings
  - Mild and persistent anemia, hypochromia with microcytosis and target cells; red blood cell count normal or elevated
  - Similar findings in one of patient's parents
  - Patient often of Mediterranean, African, or southern Chinese ancestry
  - Elevated hemoglobin A_2 and hemoglobin F

- ■ Differential Diagnosis
  - Iron deficiency anemia
  - Other hemoglobinopathies
  - Sideroblastic anemia
  - Alpha-thalassemia

- ■ Treatment
  - Oral folic acid supplementation
  - Avoidance of medicinal iron or oxidative agents
  - Red blood cell transfusions during pregnancy or stress (intercurrent illness) if hemoglobin falls below 9 g/dL

Alpha-Thalassemia Trait

- ■ Essentials of Diagnosis
    - Commonly comes to attention because of complete blood count done for other reasons
    - Family or personal history of anemia, increased frequency with African, Mediterranean, or southern Chinese ancestry
    - Microcytosis out of proportion to anemia; occasional target cells and acanthocytes on smear; normal iron studies; normal hemoglobin electrophoresis
    - No increase in hemoglobin A_2 or hemoglobin F
    - Diagnosis of exclusion in patient with modest anemia (definitive diagnosis depends on hemoglobin gene mapping)

- ■ Differential Diagnosis
    - Iron deficiency anemia
    - Other hemoglobinopathies
    - Sideroblastic anemia
    - Beta-thalassemia minor
    - Anemia of chronic disease

- ■ Treatment
    - Oral folic acid supplementation
    - Avoidance of medical iron or oxidative agents
    - Red blood cell transfusions during pregnancy or stress (intercurrent illness) if hemoglobin falls below 9 g/dL

5

Sideroblastic Anemia

- ■ Essentials of Diagnosis
  - Modest anemia; dimorphic (ie, normal and hypochromic) red blood cell population on smear
  - Elevated serum iron with high percentage saturation; marrow is diagnostic with ringed sideroblasts (iron deposits encircling red blood cell precursor nuclei)
  - Occasional history of exposure to offending drugs, lead, or alcoholism present, but most cases are idiopathic
  - Minority progress to acute leukemia

- ■ Differential Diagnosis
  - Iron deficiency anemia
  - Anemia of chronic disease
  - Thalassemia

- ■ Treatment
  - Remove offending toxin if present
  - Chelation therapy for lead toxicity
  - Pyridoxine 200 mg/d occasionally helpful
  - Most do not respond to erythropoietin

Vitamin B$_{12}$ Deficiency

- ■ Essentials of Diagnosis
    - Nonspecific gastrointestinal symptoms
    - Constant, symmetric numbness and tingling of the feet; later, poor balance and dementia manifest
    - Pallor, mild jaundice, decreased vibratory and position sense
    - Pancytopenia with oval macrocytes and hypersegmented neutrophils, increased MCV, megaloblastic bone marrow; serum vitamin B$_{12}$ < 100 ng/mL; positive Schilling test
    - Neurologic manifestations occur without anemia in occasional cases
    - Occasional previous history of total gastrectomy, bowel resection, Crohn's disease, or autoimmune endocrinopathies (eg, diabetes, hypothyroidism)

- ■ Differential Diagnosis
    - Folic acid deficiency
    - Myelodysplastic syndromes
    - Occasional hemolytic anemias with megaloblastoid red cell precursors in marrow
    - Infiltrative granulomatous or malignant processes causing pancytopenia
    - Hypersplenism

- ■ Treatment
    - Vitamin B$_{12}$ 100 μg intramuscularly daily during first week, then weekly for 1 month
    - Lifelong vitamin B$_{12}$ 100 μg intramuscularly every month thereafter
    - Hypokalemia may complicate early therapy

Folic Acid Deficiency

■ **Essentials of Diagnosis**

- Nonspecific gastrointestinal symptoms without neurologic complaints in a patient with malnutrition, often related to alcoholism
- Pallor, mild jaundice
- Pancytopenia, but counts not as low as in vitamin B_{12} deficiency; oval macrocytosis and hypersegmented neutrophils; megaloblastic marrow; normal vitamin B_{12} levels
- Red blood cell folate < 150 ng/mL diagnostic

■ **Differential Diagnosis**

- Vitamin B_{12} deficiency
- Myelodysplastic syndromes
- Infectious or malignant marrow infiltrative processes
- Hypersplenism

■ **Treatment**

- Exclude vitamin B_{12} deficiency prior to therapy
- Oral folic acid supplementation

Pure Red Cell Aplasia

- ■ Essentials of Diagnosis
    - Autoimmune disease in which IgG antibody attacks erythroid precursors
    - Lassitude, malaise; nonspecific examination except for pallor
    - Severe anemia with normal red blood cell morphology; myeloid and platelet lines unaffected; low or absent reticulocyte count
    - Reduced or absent erythroid precursors in normocellular marrow
    - Rare associations with systemic lupus erythematosus, chronic lymphocytic leukemia, non-Hodgkin's lymphoma and thymoma

- ■ Differential Diagnosis
    - Aplastic anemia
    - Myelodysplastic syndromes
    - Drug-induced red cell aplasia

- ■ Treatment
    - Evaluate for underlying disease
    - Immunosuppressive therapy with prednisone, cyclophosphamide, antithymocyte globulin
    - High-dose intravenous immune globulin in selected patients

5

Aplastic Anemia

- **Essentials of Diagnosis**
  - Lassitude, fatigue, malaise, other nonspecific symptoms
  - Pallor, purpura, mucosal bleeding, petechiae, infection
  - Pancytopenia with normal cellular morphology; hypocellular bone marrow with fatty infiltration
  - History of exposure to an offending drug or radiation

- **Differential Diagnosis**
  - Myelofibrosis
  - Acute leukemia
  - Hypersplenism
  - Infection or tumor infiltrating marrow
  - AIDS
  - Systemic lupus erythematosus (SLE)

- **Treatment**
  - Allogeneic bone marrow transplantation for patients under age 30
  - Antithymocyte globulin, cyclosporine if transplant not feasible
  - Oral androgens may be of benefit
  - If SLE associated, plasmapheresis and corticosteroids effective
  - Avoid transfusions if possible in patients who may be transplant candidates; otherwise, red blood cells and platelet transfusions, G-CSF or GM-CSF as necessary

Autoimmune Hemolytic Anemia

- **Essentials of Diagnosis**
  - Acquired anemia caused by IgG autoantibody
  - Fatigue, malaise in many; occasional abdominal or back pain
  - Pallor, jaundice, splenomegaly on examination
  - Persistent anemia with spherocytes and reticulocytosis; elevated indirect bilirubin and serum LDH
  - Positive Coombs test
  - Exposure to offending drugs or underlying autoimmune disorder may be present

- **Differential Diagnosis**
  - Hemoglobinopathy
  - Spherocytosis
  - Nonspherocytic hemolytic anemia
  - Sideroblastic anemia
  - Cold agglutinin disease

- **Treatment**
  - Oral high-dose prednisone
  - Caution in use of red blood cell transfusions (difficulty cross-matching may lead to incompatible transfusion)
  - Splenectomy if no response to prednisone after 1–2 months or if high doses required to maintain remission
  - Immunosuppressive regimens or intravenous immune globulin for treatment failures

5

Hemolytic Transfusion Reactions

- **Essentials of Diagnosis**
    - Chills and fever during blood transfusion
    - Pain in back, chest, or abdomen; dark urine
    - Associated with vascular collapse, renal failure, and disseminated intravascular coagulation
    - Hemolysis, hemoglobinuria, and severe anemia

5

- **Differential Diagnosis**
    - Leukoagglutination reaction
    - IgA deficiency
    - Myocardial infarction
    - Acute abdomen due to other causes
    - Septicemia

- **Treatment**
    - Stop transfusion immediately
    - Hydration and intravenous mannitol to prevent renal failure

Hereditary Spherocytosis

- **Essentials of Diagnosis**
    - Malaise, abdominal discomfort in symptomatic patients
    - Jaundice, splenomegaly
    - Variable anemia with spherocytosis and reticulocytosis; elevated MCHC; increased osmotic fragility test, negative Coombs test
    - Family history of anemia, jaundice, splenectomy

- **Differential Diagnosis**
    - Autoimmune hemolytic anemia
    - Hemoglobin C disease
    - Alcoholism
    - Burns

- **Treatment**
    - Oral folic acid supplementation
    - Pneumococcal vaccination if splenectomy contemplated
    - Splenectomy for symptomatic patients

Paroxysmal Nocturnal Hemoglobinuria

- **Essentials of Diagnosis**
    - Episodic red-brown urine, especially on first morning specimen
    - Variable anemia with or without leukopenia, thrombocytopenia; reticulocytosis; positive urine hemosiderin, elevated serum LDH; positive sucrose hemolysis test
    - Diagnosis confirmed by Ham's (acidified serum) test
    - Iron deficiency often concurrent
    - History of unusual or unexpected thrombotic event, especially venous

- **Differential Diagnosis**
    - Hemolytic anemias
    - Pancytopenia due to other causes

- **Treatment**
    - Prednisone for moderate to severe cases
    - Oral iron replacement if iron-deficient
    - Allogeneic bone marrow transplantation for severe cases

Sickle Cell Anemia

- ■ Essentials of Diagnosis
  - Recurrent attacks of fever and pain in arms, legs, or abdomen starting in early childhood
  - Splenomegaly in early childhood *only;* jaundice, pallor; adults are functionally asplenic
  - Anemia and elevated reticulocyte count with irreversibly sickled cells on peripheral smear; elevated indirect bilirubin, LDH; positive sickling test; hemoglobin S and F on electrophoresis
  - Positive family history and lifelong history of hemolytic anemia

- ■ Differential Diagnosis
  - Other hemoglobinopathies
  - Acute rheumatic fever
  - Osteomyelitis
  - Acute abdomen due to any cause
  - If hematuria present, renal stone or tumor

- ■ Treatment
  - Chronic oral folic acid supplementation
  - Hydration and analgesics
  - Hydroxyurea for patients with frequent crises
  - Partial exchange transfusions for intractable vaso-occlusive crises
  - Transfusion for hemolytic or aplastic crises and during third trimester of pregnancy
  - Pneumococcal vaccination
  - Genetic counseling

Hemoglobin SC Disease

- **Essentials of Diagnosis**
  - Recurrent attacks of abdominal, joint, or bone pain
  - Splenomegaly, retinopathy (similar to diabetes)
  - Mild anemia, reticulocytosis, and few sickle cells on smear with many target cells; positive sickle test; 50% hemoglobin C, 50% hemoglobin S on electrophoresis
  - In situ thrombi of pulmonary artery, venous sinus of brain may cause stroke, mimic pulmonary emboli

- **Differential Diagnosis**
  - Sickle cell anemia
  - Sickle thalassemia
  - Hemoglobin C disease
  - Cirrhosis
  - Pulmonary embolism

- **Treatment**
  - No specific therapy for most patients
  - Increased risk for thrombotic events, bone infarctions, and retinopathy

Hemoglobin S-Thalassemia Disease

- ■ Essentials of Diagnosis
  - Recurrent attacks of abdominal, joint, or bone pain
  - Splenomegaly
  - Mild to moderate anemia with low MCV; reticulocytosis; few sickle cells on smear with many target cells; increased hemoglobin A_2 by electrophoresis distinguishes from sickle cell disease

- ■ Differential Diagnosis
  - Sickle cell anemia
  - Hemoglobin C disease
  - Hemoglobin SC disease
  - Cirrhosis

- ■ Treatment
  - Chronic oral folic acid supplementation
  - Acute therapy as in sickle cell anemia

Microangiopathic Hemolytic Anemia

- ■ Essentials of Diagnosis
  - Malaise, mucosal or cutaneous bleeding, fleeting neurologic complaints
  - Fever, mild jaundice, petechiae, neurologic abnormalities
  - Severe anemia with fragmented red blood cells on smear (schistocytes, helmet cells); thrombocytopenia, greatly elevated serum LDH, abnormal renal function tests
  - Associations with exposure to offending drugs, peripartum period, dysenteric disease, or AIDS
  - Thrombotic thrombocytopenic purpura (TTP) is the most important microangiopathic hemolytic anemia; associated with fever, thrombocytopenia, neurologic and renal abnormalities

- ■ Causes
  - TTP
  - Malignant hypertension
  - Metastatic adenocarcinoma
  - Preeclampsia-eclampsia
  - Vasculitides
  - Disseminated intravascular coagulation
  - Mechanical valve hemolysis

- ■ Treatment
  - Early therapy with plasmapheresis for TTP
  - Splenectomy, high-dose corticosteroids, intravenous dextran for plasmapheresis failures
  - Avoid platelet transfusions that may precipitate thrombotic event

Acute Leukemia

■ **Essentials of Diagnosis**
  • Fairly abrupt onset of fever, weakness, malaise, bleeding, bone or joint pain, infection
  • Pallor, fever, petechiae; lymphadenopathy, splenomegaly unusual
  • Leukocytosis or pancytopenia; immature, abnormal white cells in peripheral blood and bone marrow
  • Abnormal cells are either lymphoblasts (ALL) or myeloblasts (AML)

■ **Differential Diagnosis**
  • Aplastic anemia
  • Idiopathic thrombocytopenia purpura
  • Infectious mononucleosis
  • Hodgkin's or non-Hodgkin's lymphoma
  • Pertussis
  • Metastatic malignancy to bone marrow
  • Tuberculosis
  • Paroxysmal nocturnal hemoglobinuria

■ **Treatment**
  • Aggressive combination chemotherapy with specific drugs dictated by cell type
  • Allogeneic or autologous bone marrow transplantations for patients in remission who are less than 55–60 years of age

Chronic Myelogenous Leukemia

- ■ Essentials of Diagnosis
    - Symptoms variable; often suspected because of blood count done for unrelated reasons
    - Painless splenomegaly common; sternal tenderness in some
    - Leukocytosis, immature white cells in peripheral blood and bone marrow; thrombocytosis, eosinophilia, basophilia common
    - Low leukocyte alkaline phosphatase level, markedly elevated serum vitamin B_{12} markers
    - Philadelphia chromosome present in 95% of cases

- ■ Differential Diagnosis
    - Leukemoid reactions associated with infection, inflammation, or cancer
    - Other myeloproliferative disorders

- ■ Treatment
    - Myelosuppressive therapy for symptoms of acute phase
    - Hydroxyurea, alpha interferon, busulfan, cyclophosphamide
    - Allogeneic bone marrow transplantation during chronic phase for patients who are under 55 years of age
    - Leukapheresis for leukocytosis associated with hyperviscosity syndromes

Chronic Lymphocytic Leukemia

- ■ Essentials of Diagnosis
  - Fatigue in some; most asymptomatic
  - Pallor, lymphadenopathy, variable hepatosplenomegaly
  - Lymphocytosis > 15,000/µL or higher, with some counts up to 1,000,000/µL; morphologically mature cells
  - Coombs-positive hemolytic anemia, thrombocytopenia, hypogammaglobulinemia sometimes associated with poorer prognosis

- ■ Differential Diagnosis
  - Infectious mononucleosis
  - Lymphoma in leukemic stage
  - Pertussis

- ■ Treatment
  - Oral chlorambucil and prednisone for symptomatic leukocytosis, anemia, or thrombocytopenia
  - Splenectomy for autoimmune hemolytic anemia or immune thrombocytopenia
  - Fludarabine, cladribine for refractory disease

Polycythemia Vera

- ■ Essentials of Diagnosis
  - Acquired myeloproliferative disorder with overproduction of all three hematopoietic cell lines
  - Malaise, pruritus with warm exposure to skin, tinnitus, blurred vision
  - Plethoric facies, splenomegaly
  - Elevated hematocrit; leukocytosis with basophilia and thrombocytosis common; elevated total red blood cell mass, normal P_{O_2}
  - Increased serum vitamin B_{12}, leukocyte alkaline phosphatase levels usually elevated; high serum uric acid
  - Patients predisposed to both bleeding and thrombosis

- ■ Differential Diagnosis
  - Hypoxia (pulmonary or cardiac disease, high altitude)
  - Carboxyhemoglobin (tobacco use)
  - Certain hemoglobinopathies
  - Erythropoietin-secreting tumors
  - Cystic renal disease
  - Spurious erythrocytosis with decreased plasma volume and normal red cell mass (diuretic use)
  - Other myeloproliferative disorders

- ■ Treatment
  - Phlebotomy to lower hematocrit to less than 45%
  - Myelosuppressive therapy for patients with high phlebotomy requirements, intractable pruritus, or marked thrombocytosis
  - Avoidance of medicinal iron
  - Aspirin 325 mg/d
  - Hydroxyurea, busulfan, alpha interferon

Myelofibrosis

- **Essentials of Diagnosis**
  - Fatigue, abdominal discomfort, bleeding, bone pain
  - Massive splenomegaly, variable hepatomegaly
  - Anemia, variable leukocytosis; leukoerythroblastic peripheral smear with teardrop poikilocytosis and giant platelets
  - "Dry tap" on bone marrow aspiration

- **Differential Diagnosis**
  - Chronic myelocytic leukemia
  - Other myeloproliferative disorders
  - Hemolytic anemias
  - Hodgkin's disease
  - Metastatic cancer of bone marrow
  - Hairy cell leukemia

- **Treatment**
  - Red blood cell transfusion support
  - Androgenic steroids may decrease transfusion requirements
  - Splenectomy for painful splenomegaly, severe thrombocytopenia, or extraordinary red blood cell requirements
  - Alpha interferon or erythropoietin (or both together) may be of benefit in selected patients

5

Hairy Cell Leukemia

- **Essentials of Diagnosis**
  - Fatigue, abdominal pain, infection
  - Pallor, massive splenomegaly, variable hepatomegaly, rare lymphadenopathy
  - Pancytopenia, "hairy cell" morphology of leukocytes in periphery and marrow
  - "Dry tap" on bone marrow aspiration; diagnostic tartrate-resistant acid phosphatase (TRAP) stain

- **Differential Diagnosis**
  - Chronic lymphocytic leukemia
  - Waldenström's macroglobulinemia
  - Non-Hodgkin's lymphoma

- **Treatment**
  - Cladribine, pentostatin
  - Splenectomy for severe cytopenias or recurrent infections

Myelodysplastic Syndromes

■ Essentials of Diagnosis
  - Begins as refractory anemia with symptoms and signs thereof
  - Cytopenias and macrocytosis common as disease progresses, with abnormal neutrophil morphology (eg, Pelger-Huët anomaly) and giant platelets, and finally peripheral blasts
  - Hypercellular bone marrow, abnormal morphology (eg, ringed sideroblasts early)
  - Previous chemotherapy (eg, procarbazine, melphalan) predisposes

■ Differential Diagnosis
  - Acute myeloblastic leukemia
  - Anemia of chronic disease

■ Treatment
  - Poor results with low-dose chemotherapy
  - Red blood cell transfusions, erythropoietin, G-CSF and GM-CSF raise the neutrophil count and reduce the incidence of infections
  - Allogeneic bone marrow transplantation for patients less than 55 years of age

5

Non-Hodgkin's Lymphoma

- ■ Essentials of Diagnosis
  - • Painless lymphadenopathy, fever, night sweats, malaise
  - • Firm lymphadenopathy often widespread, variable hepato-splenomegaly
  - • Radiographic demonstration of lymphatic and soft tissue masses, elevated LDH
  - • Lymph node or involved extranodal tissue biopsies diagnostic

- ■ Differential Diagnosis
  - • Hodgkin's disease
  - • Lymphomatoid granulomatosis
  - • Infectious mononucleosis
  - • Cat-scratch disease
  - • Drug reaction (phenytoin)
  - • Sarcoidosis
  - • HIV disease

- ■ Treatment
  - • Staging with chest x-ray, abdominal and pelvic CT scans, bone marrow biopsy, and lumbar puncture in selected cases
  - • Treatment individualized depending on age, stage, grade, and performance status
  - • Radiation therapy for localized disease
  - • Aggressive combination chemotherapy for high-grade disease
  - • Autologous bone marrow transplantation may be effective

5

Hodgkin's Disease

- ■ Essentials of Diagnosis
  - • Fever, weight loss, night sweats, pruritus
  - • Regionally enlarged, firm, painless lymphadenopathy (often cervical); hepatosplenomegaly variable
  - • Reed-Sternberg cells in lymph node or bone marrow biopsy diagnostic

- ■ Differential Diagnosis
  - • Non-Hodgkin's lymphoma
  - • Lymphadenitis secondary to infections (tuberculosis and cat-scratch disease)
  - • Drug reaction (phenytoin)
  - • Lymphomatoid granulomatosis
  - • Sarcoidosis
  - • HIV disease

- ■ Treatment
  - • Staging with chest x-ray, CT scan of chest, abdomen, and pelvis, and bone marrow biopsy; laparotomy if results would alter therapy
  - • Radiation therapy for localized disease
  - • Aggressive combination chemotherapy for disseminated disease

Multiple Myeloma

- ■ Essentials of Diagnosis
  - Weakness, weight loss, recurrent infection, bone (especially back) pain, often with pathologic fractures
  - Pallor, bony tenderness; spleen is not enlarged
  - Anemia; elevated sedimentation rate; elevated serum calcium, renal insufficiency; normal alkaline phosphatase
  - Elevated serum globulin with monoclonal spike on protein electrophoresis
  - Immature plasma cells infiltrating bone marrow
  - Lytic bone lesions with negative bone scan

- ■ Differential Diagnosis
  - Metastatic cancer
  - Hodgkin's and non-Hodgkin's lymphomas
  - Hyperparathyroidism
  - Waldenström's macroglobulinemia
  - Benign monoclonal gammopathy
  - Primary amyloidosis
  - Aortic aneurysm

- ■ Treatment
  - Chemotherapy for renal disease and hypercalcemia
  - Melphalan and prednisone
  - Vincristine, doxorubicin, and dexamethasone if not responsive to melphalan and prednisone
  - Radiation therapy for local bone pain or pathologic fractures
  - Allogeneic or autologous bone marrow transplantation for patients under age 55

Waldenström's Macroglobulinemia

- **■ Essentials of Diagnosis**
  - Fatigue, symptoms of hyperviscosity (central nervous system involvement, bleeding, or thrombosis)
  - Variable hepatosplenomegaly and lymphadenopathy; "boxcar" retinal vein engorgement
  - Anemia with rouleau formation; monoclonal IgM paraprotein; increased serum viscosity
  - Plasmacytic lymphocytic infiltrate in marrow
  - Absence of lytic bone lesions

- **■ Differential Diagnosis**
  - Benign monoclonal gammopathy
  - Chronic lymphocytic leukemia
  - Multiple myeloma

- **■ Treatment**
  - Plasmapheresis for severe hyperviscosity (stupor or coma)
  - Chlorambucil, cyclophosphamide, fludarabine, cladribine

5

Idiopathic Thrombocytopenic Purpura

- **Essentials of Diagnosis**
  - Mucosal bleeding, easy bleeding
  - Petechiae, ecchymoses; splenomegaly rare
  - Severe thrombocytopenia, prolonged bleeding time, poor clot retraction; elevated platelet-associated IgG in 95%; normal marrow

- **Differential Diagnosis**
  - Acute leukemia
  - Myelodysplastic syndrome
  - Thrombotic microangiopathy
  - Disseminated intravascular coagulation
  - Chronic lymphocytic leukemia
  - Aplastic anemia
  - Myelofibrosis
  - Acute alcoholism
  - Drug toxicity
  - AIDS
  - Systemic lupus erythematosus

- **Treatment**
  - Prednisone
  - Splenectomy if no response to corticosteroids, or if condition persists for more than 1 year; high-dose intravenous immune globulin effective for short-lived elevation of platelets prior to surgery
  - Zidovudine if AIDS-related
  - Danazol, vincristine, vinblastine, azathioprine, or cyclophosphamide for refractory cases
  - Reserve platelet transfusion for life-threatening hemorrhages

Von Willebrand's Disease

■ Essentials of Diagnosis
- History of lifelong excessive bruising and mucosal bleeding; excessive bleeding during previous surgery, dental extraction, or childbirth
- Usually prolonged bleeding time, normal platelet count, reduced levels of factor VIII antigen or ristocetin cofactor
- Prolonged partial thromboplastin time when factor VIII coagulant levels decreased

■ Differential Diagnosis
- Glanzmann's thrombasthenia
- Waldenström's macroglobulinemia
- Drugs (aspirin)
- Hemophilias

■ Treatment
- Avoid aspirin
- Cryoprecipitate prior to dental or surgical procedures
- Factor VIII concentrates
- Desmopressin acetate for type I disease
- Tranexamic acid

Hemophilia

- ■ Essentials of Diagnosis
  - Lifelong history of bleeding in a male; usually congenital and familial
  - Slow, prolonged bleeding after minor injury or surgery; spontaneous hemarthroses common
  - Prolonged partial thromboplastin time corrected by mixing patient's plasma with a normal specimen
  - Normal factor VIII antigen; low factor VIII coagulant activity (hemophilia A) or factor IX coagulant activity (hemophilia B)

- ■ Differential Diagnosis
  - Von Willebrand's disease
  - Disseminated intravascular coagulation
  - Afibrinogenemia

- ■ Treatment
  - Avoidance of aspirin
  - Factor replacement for any bleeding with factor VIII concentrates (hemophilia A) or factor IX complex (hemophilia B)
  - Steroids or immunosuppressants if factor inhibitor develops
  - Desmopressin acetate before surgical procedures for hemophilia A

Disseminated Intravascular Coagulation

■ Essentials of Diagnosis
  • Diffuse bleeding from skin and mucous membrane or thrombosis
  • Hypofibrinogenemia, thrombocytopenia, and prolonged prothrombin time and partial thromboplastin time; elevated fibrin degradation products; microangiopathic hemolysis may be present
  • Usually caused by severe infection, tissue injury, obstetric complication, or cancer

■ Differential Diagnosis
  • Severe liver disease
  • Vitamin K deficiency
  • Primary fibrinolysis
  • Thrombocytopenia of infection
  • Thrombotic microangiopathy

■ Treatment
  • Treat underlying disorder
  • For life-threatening hemorrhage, replacement of platelets with transfusion or fibrinogen with cryoprecipitate
  • Heparin in selected cases
  • Aminocaproic acid or tranexamic acid in cases refractory to heparin and platelets; discontinue heparin before starting aminocaproic acid

5

Circulating Anticoagulants

- **Essentials of Diagnosis**
  - Ecchymoses or mucosal bleeding, especially gastrointestinal; hemarthroses less common than in hemophilia
  - Elevated partial thromboplastin time does not correct with mixing study
  - Reduced factor VIII coagulant activity

- **Differential Diagnosis**
  - Macroglobulinemia
  - Multiple myeloma
  - Cryoglobulinemia
  - Von Willebrand's disease
  - Hemophilia
  - Systemic lupus erythematosus

- **Treatment**
  - Prednisone, plasmapheresis, cyclophosphamide
  - Factor VIII replacement

5

6

Rheumatologic & Autoimmune Disorders

Degenerative Joint Disease (Osteoarthritis)

- **Essentials of Diagnosis**
    - Progressive degeneration of articular cartilage and hypertrophy of bone at the articular margins
    - Affects almost all joints, especially weight-bearing and frequently used joints
    - May be primary (idiopathic) or secondary to trauma, metabolic abnormality, or other articular disease
    - Primary degenerative joint disease most commonly affects the distal interphalangeal joints (Heberden's nodes), hips, and first carpometacarpal joints
    - Pain relieved by rest; morning stiffness brief; articular inflammation minimal
    - Radiographs reveal narrowing of the joint spaces, osteophytes, increased density of subchondral bone, bony cysts

- **Differential Diagnosis**
    - Rheumatoid arthritis
    - Seronegative spondyloarthropathies
    - Crystal-induced arthritides
    - Metastatic neoplasm
    - Osteoporosis
    - Multiple myeloma

- **Treatment**
    - Weight reduction
    - Exercises to strengthen muscles around affected joints
    - Aspirin, other NSAIDs (eg, ibuprofen, 600 mg three times daily)
    - Intra-articular corticosteroid injection (eg, triamcinolone, 10–40 mg) in selected cases
    - Surgery for severely affected joints, especially hip

Gout

- ■ **Essentials of Diagnosis**
    - Spectrum of disease, including recurrent arthritic attacks, appearance of tophi, nephropathy, and uric acid nephrolithiasis
    - Recurring acute arthritis typically nocturnal and usually monarticular; may be polyarticular with repeated attacks
    - Affects first metatarsophalangeal joint (podagra), mid foot, ankle, knees, wrist, elbow; hips and shoulders spared
    - Hyperuricemia may be primary (caused by overproduction (10%) or underexcretion (90%) of uric acid) or secondary to diuretic use, cytotoxic drugs, myeloproliferative disorders, multiple myeloma, hemoglobinopathies, chronic renal disease, hypothyroidism
    - After long periods of untreated hyperuricemia, tophi (monosodium urate deposits with an associated foreign body reaction) develop in subcutaneous tissues, bone, cartilage, joints, and other tissues
    - Identification of weakly negative birefringent, needle-like, urate crystals in joint fluid or tophi is diagnostic

- ■ **Differential Diagnosis**
    - Cellulitis
    - Septic arthritis
    - Pseudogout
    - Rheumatoid arthritis
    - Calcium oxalate deposition disease
    - Chronic lead intoxication (saturnine gout)

- ■ **Treatment**
    - Treat the acute arthritis first and the hyperuricemia later, if at all
    - For acute attacks: dramatic therapeutic response to NSAIDs (eg, indomethacin, 50 mg three times daily), colchicine, intra-articular or systemic corticosteroids
    - For chronic prophylaxis in patients with frequent acute attacks, tophaceous deposits, or renal damage: allopurinol (decreases uric acid synthesis by inhibiting xanthine oxidase) and probenecid (uricosuric agent) with concomitant colchicine
    - Avoid thiazides and loop diuretics, which inhibit renal excretion of uric acid

Chondrocalcinosis & Pseudogout (Calcium Pyrophosphate Dihydrate Deposition Disease)

- **■ Essentials of Diagnosis**
  - Chondrocalcinosis refers to the presence of calcium-containing salts in articular cartilage
  - Acute, recurrent, and rarely chronic arthritis usually involving large joints (especially knees and wrists) and almost always accompanied by chondrocalcinosis of the affected joints
  - May be hereditary, idiopathic, or associated with metabolic disorders, including hemochromatosis, hyperparathyroidism, ochronosis, diabetes mellitus, hypothyroidism, Wilson's disease, and gout
  - Identification of calcium pyrophosphate rhomboid-shaped crystals (positively birefringent) in the joint fluid is diagnostic
  - Radiographs may reveal chondrocalcinosis or signs of degenerative joint disease

- **■ Differential Diagnosis**
  - Gout
  - Calcium phosphate disease (hydroxyapatite arthropathy)
  - Calcium oxalate deposition disease
  - Degenerative joint disease
  - Rheumatoid arthritis

- **■ Treatment**
  - Treat underlying disease if present
  - Aspirin, other NSAIDs (eg, indomethacin, 50 mg three times daily)
  - Intra-articular injection of corticosteroids (eg, triamcinolone, 10–40 mg)
  - Colchicine, 0.6 mg twice daily, occasionally useful for prophylaxis

Rheumatoid Arthritis

- **Essentials of Diagnosis**
  - Symmetric polyarthritis of peripheral joints with pain, tenderness, and swelling of affected joints; morning stiffness common, lasting more than an hour
  - Chronic, persistent synovitis with formation of pannus which erodes cartilage, bone, ligaments, and tendons
  - Joint deformities may develop; proximal interphalangeal and metacarpophalangeal joints frequently involved; ulnar deviation of digits common
  - Rheumatoid factor usually present
  - Extra-articular manifestations include subcutaneous nodules, vasculitis, pericarditis, pleural effusion (low in glucose), lymphadenopathy, scleritis, sicca syndrome, Felty's syndrome (splenomegaly with leukopenia); usually in strongly seropositive patients
  - Radiographic findings include juxta-articular and sometimes generalized osteoporosis, narrowing of the joint spaces, and bony erosions

- **Differential Diagnosis**
  - Systemic lupus erythematosus
  - Degenerative joint disease
  - Gout or pseudogout
  - Lyme disease
  - Polymyalgia rheumatica

- **Treatment**
  - Unless contraindicated, aspirin (1 g four times daily) is first-line therapy
  - NSAIDs (eg, ibuprofen, 800 mg three times daily) equally effective with less gastrointestinal toxicity
  - Hydroxychloroquine and minocycline have modest efficacy for mild disease
  - Methotrexate, gold salts, azathioprine, penicillamine, corticosteroids, and experimental therapies may be used in severe disease
  - Surgery for severely affected joints

Adult-Onset Still's Disease (Systemic-Onset Form of Juvenile Rheumatoid Arthritis)

- ■ Essentials of Diagnosis
  - Systemic form of juvenile rheumatoid arthritis (Still's disease) can occur in adults
  - High spiking fevers may antedate arthritis by months; no arthritis in some cases
  - Polyarthritis or oligoarthritis usually affects the proximal inter-phalangeal and metacarpophalangeal joints, wrists, knees, hips and shoulders
  - Characteristic evanescent, salmon-colored, maculopapular rash involving the trunk and extremities
  - Systemic manifestations including hepatosplenomegaly, lymphadenopathy, pleuropericarditis, anemia, and leukocytosis

- ■ Differential Diagnosis
  - Leukemia or lymphoma
  - Arthritis associated with inflammatory bowel disease
  - Chronic infection
  - Vasculitis
  - Systemic lupus erythematosus
  - Lyme disease

- ■ Treatment
  - Unless contraindicated, aspirin (1 g four times daily); often dramatically reduces fever
  - NSAIDs (eg, ibuprofen, 800 mg three times daily)
  - Corticosteroids, gold, hydroxychloroquine, penicillamine, methotrexate, azathioprine, and other immunosuppressive agents have been used

Systemic Lupus Erythematosus

- ■ Essentials of Diagnosis
    - Multisystem, inflammatory, autoimmune disorder
    - Predominantly in young women with periods of exacerbation and remission
    - Four or more of the following 11 criteria must be present: malar ("butterfly") rash, discoid rash, photosensitivity, oral ulcers, arthritis, serositis, renal disease, neurologic disease, hematologic disorders, positive antinuclear antibody (ANA), and immunologic abnormalities (eg, antibody to native DNA or false-positive serologic test for syphilis)
    - Also associated with fever, myositis, alopecia, myocarditis, pericarditis, vasculitis, lymphadenopathy, conjunctivitis, venous or arterial thrombosis, glomerulonephritis, sicca complex
    - Syndrome may be drug-induced (especially procainamide, hydralazine); brain and kidney spared

- ■ Differential Diagnosis
    - Rheumatoid arthritis
    - Vasculitis
    - Sjögren's syndrome
    - Systemic sclerosis
    - Endocarditis

- ■ Treatment
    - Aspirin (1 g four times daily); other NSAIDs (eg, ibuprofen, 800 mg three times daily)
    - Corticosteroids, hydroxychloroquine, cyclophosphamide, azathioprine in aggressive disease
    - Withdraw offending agent if drug-induced
    - Avoid sun exposure

Systemic Sclerosis (Scleroderma)

- **Essentials of Diagnosis**
  - Diffuse systemic sclerosis (20% of patients) with diffuse fibrotic changes of the skin and internal organ systems; Raynaud's phenomenon and polyarthralgia typical; associated with intestinal hypomotility, pulmonary fibrosis, myopericarditis, hypertension, renal failure
  - Limited systemic sclerosis (80% of patients) associated with CREST syndrome (calcinosis cutis, Raynaud's phenomenon, esophageal hypomotility, sclerodactyly, and telangiectasia); skin tightening limited to distal extremities; lower risk of renal disease, later risk of pulmonary hypertension and biliary cirrhosis; overall better prognosis
  - ANA frequently useful; anticentromere antibody in 1% of patients with diffuse scleroderma, 50% of patients with CREST syndrome; antitopoisomerase I (Scl-70) one-third in diffuse systemic sclerosis, 20% in CREST syndrome

- **Differential Diagnosis**
  - Eosinophilic fasciitis
  - Eosinophilia-myalgia syndrome
  - Overlap syndromes
  - Graft-versus-host disease
  - Amyloidosis
  - Systemic lupus erythematosus

- **Treatment**
  - Penicillamine, 250 mg/d
  - Corticosteroids not helpful
  - Warm clothing, smoking cessation, and nifedipine for Raynaud's phenomenon; intravenous iloprost may be helpful for digital ulcers
  - H_2 receptor antagonists or omeprazole for esophageal reflux

Overlap Syndromes (Mixed Connective Tissue Disease & Undifferentiated Connective Tissue Syndrome)

- ### Essentials of Diagnosis
  - Clinical features of more than one disease (SLE, systemic sclerosis, polymyositis, and rheumatoid arthritis)
  - Sicca complex (xerostomia, xerophthalmia, dry cough) and myositis in virtually all patients
  - Associated with Raynaud's phenomenon, pulmonary fibrosis, polyarthritis, pericarditis, myocarditis, esophageal hypomotility, glomerulonephritis
  - Presence of a specific antibody to ribonuclear protein (RNP)
  - May evolve to one predominant disease over time

- ### Differential Diagnosis
  - Systemic lupus erythematosus
  - Systemic sclerosis
  - Polymyositis
  - Sjögren's syndrome
  - Rheumatoid arthritis
  - Eosinophilic fasciitis
  - Graft-versus-host disease

- ### Treatment
  - Aspirin (1 g four times daily); other NSAIDs (eg, ibuprofen, 800 mg three times daily)
  - Corticosteroids in moderate doses often effective
  - Symptomatic relief of dryness with artificial tears, chewing gum, sialagogues, frequent sips of water
  - Warm clothing, smoking cessation, and nifedipine for Raynaud's phenomenon

Polymyositis-Dermatomyositis

- ■ Essentials of Diagnosis
  - Bilateral proximal muscle weakness
  - Periorbital edema and a purplish (heliotrope) rash over the upper eyelids in many
  - Violaceous, occasionally scaly papules overlying the dorsal surface of the interphalangeal joints of the hands (Gottron's papules)
  - Serum CK elevated; ANA in most; anti-Jo-1 antibodies in the subset of patients who have associated interstitial lung disease
  - Muscle biopsy usually diagnostic
  - May be associated with rheumatoid arthritis, SLE, scleroderma, mixed connective tissue disease; increased incidence of malignancy, especially in older patients

- ■ Differential Diagnosis
  - Hypothyroidism
  - Endocrine myopathies (eg, hyperthyroidism)
  - Polymyalgia rheumatica
  - Myasthenia gravis
  - Eaton-Lambert syndrome
  - Muscular dystrophy
  - Rhabdomyolysis
  - Parasitic myositis
  - Drug-induced myopathies (eg, corticosteroids, alcohol, colchicine, lovastatin, zidovudine, hydroxychloroquine, tryptophan)
  - Inclusion body myositis

- ■ Treatment
  - Corticosteroids
  - Methotrexate
  - Azathioprine
  - Intravenous immune globulin for dermatomyositis

Sjögren's Syndrome

- ■ Essentials of Diagnosis
  - • Destruction of exocrine glands leading to mucosal and conjunctival dryness
  - • Dry mouth (xerostomia) and dry eyes (keratoconjunctivitis sicca), decreased tear production, parotid enlargement, severe dental caries, loss of taste and smell
  - • Occasionally associated with nephritis, vasculitis, pancreatitis, pleuritis, neuropsychiatric dysfunction, polyneuropathy, interstitial pneumonitis, thyroid disease, cardiac conduction defects
  - • Over 50% have cytoplasmic antibodies, anti-Ro (SS-A), and anti-La (SS-B)
  - • Decreased lacrimation measured by Schirmer's filter paper test; biopsy of minor salivary glands of lower lip confirms diagnosis
  - • May be observed in patients with rheumatoid arthritis, SLE, primary biliary cirrhosis, systemic sclerosis, polymyositis, polyarteritis, or interstitial pulmonary fibrosis; increased incidence of lymphoma and Waldenström's macroglobulinemia

- ■ Differential Diagnosis
  - • Sicca complex associated with other autoimmune diseases
  - • Sarcoidosis

- ■ Treatment
  - • Symptomatic relief of dryness with artificial tears, chewing gum, sialagogues
  - • Anticholinergic drug use
  - • Meticulous care of teeth and avoidance of sugar-containing candies
  - • Corticosteroids or cyclophosphamide for extraglandular manifestations

Polyarteritis Nodosa

- ■ Essentials of Diagnosis
  - Fever, hypertension, abdominal pain, arthralgias, myalgias
  - Cotton-wool spots, microaneurysms, pericarditis, myocarditis, palpable purpura, livedo reticularis, mononeuritis multiplex; usually spares the lung
  - Individual patients may have any variation of the above symptoms and signs
  - Elevation of sedimentation rate in most patients; serologic evidence of hepatitis B or hepatitis C in 30–50%
  - Inflammation of small- and medium-sized arteries on biopsy specimens
  - Diagnosis confirmed by visceral angiography

- ■ Differential Diagnosis
  - Wegener's granulomatosis
  - Churg-Strauss vasculitis
  - Hypersensitivity vasculitis
  - Infective endocarditis
  - Essential mixed cryoglobulinemia
  - Cholesterol atheroembolic disease

- ■ Treatment
  - Corticosteroids alone produce temporary remission
  - Addition of cyclophosphamide or azathioprine preferable

Polymyalgia Rheumatica & Giant Cell Arteritis

■ Essentials of Diagnosis

- Polymyalgia rheumatica characterized by pain and stiffness, not weakness, of the shoulder and pelvic girdle lasting 1 month or more without other explanation
- Associated with fever, minimal joint swelling, elevated sedimentation rate, and rapid response (usually within 72 hours) to low-dose prednisone
- Patients usually over age 50
- Giant cell (temporal) arteritis is a vasculitis affecting medium- and large-sized vessels; frequently coexists with polymyalgia rheumatica
- Headache, transient or permanent blindness, jaw claudication, temporal artery tenderness; aortic regurgitation, mononeuritis multiplex less common
- Diagnosis confirmed by 5 cm temporal artery biopsy (reliable within 1–2 weeks after starting prednisone)

■ Differential Diagnosis

- Multiple myeloma
- Chronic infection, eg, endocarditis, visceral abscess
- Neoplasm
- Rheumatoid arthritis
- Hypothyroidism
- Polymyositis
- Headache due to other cause

■ Treatment

- Prednisone 10–20 mg/d for polymyalgia rheumatica
- Prednisone 60 mg/d immediately on suspicion of temporal arteritis

Churg-Strauss Vasculitis
(Allergic Granulomatosis & Angiitis)

- **Essentials of Diagnosis**
  - Granulomatous vasculitis of small- and medium-sized arteries
  - Occurs in patients with asthma or allergic rhinitis
  - Associated with transient pulmonary infiltrates, palpable purpura, arthritis, hypertension, mononeuritis multiplex, glomerulonephritis

- **Differential Diagnosis**
  - Wegener's granulomatosis
  - Eosinophilic pneumonia
  - Polyarteritis nodosa

- **Treatment**
  - Corticosteroids
  - Cyclophosphamide

Hypersensitivity Vasculitis

- Essentials of Diagnosis
  - Leukocytoclastic vasculitis of small blood vessels
  - Palpable purpura the predominant feature
  - Secondary to drugs, neoplasms, connective tissue disorders, congenital complement deficiency, serum sickness, viral or bacterial infection
  - On occasion associated with fever, arthralgias, abdominal pain with or without gastrointestinal bleeding, pulmonary infiltrates, kidney involvement with hematuria

- Differential Diagnosis
  - Polyarteritis nodosa
  - Henoch-Schönlein purpura
  - Mixed cryoglobulinemia
  - Meningococcemia

- Treatment
  - Treat underlying disease if present
  - Discontinue offending drug
  - Corticosteroids

Wegener's Granulomatosis

- ■ Essentials of Diagnosis
    - Vasculitis associated with glomerulonephritis and necrotizing granulomas of upper and lower respiratory tract
    - Ninety percent of patients present with upper or lower respiratory tract symptoms including perforation of nasal septum, chronic sinusitis, otitis media, mastoiditis, cough, dyspnea, hemoptysis
    - Proptosis, scleritis, arthritis, purpura, or neuropathy may also be present
    - Chest film may reveal large nodular densities; urinalysis can show hematuria, red cell casts
    - Positive antineutrophil cytoplasmic antibody (usually C-ANCA cytoplasmic pattern) seen in 90%; nasal, lung, or renal biopsy can confirm the diagnosis, though the latter is seldom specific
    - Increased risk of bladder cancer and lymphoma

- ■ Differential Diagnosis
    - Polyarteritis nodosa
    - Churg-Strauss vasculitis
    - Goodpasture's syndrome
    - Takayasu's arteritis
    - Microscopic polyarteritis

- ■ Treatment
    - Corticosteroids
    - Cyclophosphamide, methotrexate
    - Trimethoprim-sulfamethoxazole may be effective in mild disease

6

Cryoglobulinemia

- **Essentials of Diagnosis**
  - Vasculitis, palpable purpura, glomerulonephritis, and peripheral neuropathy, usually in women
  - Associated with polyarthralgias, abdominal pain, cold-induced urticaria, hepatosplenomegaly, leg ulcers, abnormal liver function tests, Raynaud's phenomenon
  - Due to precipitation of protein at < 37°C
  - Monoclonal cryoglobulins in multiple myeloma, macroglobulinemia, or lymphoproliferative disorders
  - Mixed cryoglobulins in patients with connective tissue disease, infectious mononucleosis, cytomegalovirus, infective endocarditis, Lyme disease, syphilis, parasitic infection, sarcoidosis
  - If none of these causes can be identified, the disorder is termed essential mixed cryoglobulinemia; association with hepatitis C is common, however

- **Differential Diagnosis**
  - Lymphoproliferative disease
  - Poststreptococcal glomerulonephritis
  - Infective endocarditis
  - Polyarteritis nodosa
  - Henoch-Schönlein purpura

- **Treatment**
  - Corticosteroids
  - Immunosuppressive agents (eg, cyclophosphamide)
  - Plasmapheresis
  - Patients with hepatitis C may respond to interferon-alfa

Takayasu's Arteritis ("Pulseless Disease")

- ■ Essentials of Diagnosis
  - Large-vessel vasculitis involving the aortic arch and its major branches
  - Most frequent in young women of Asian descent
  - Associated with myalgias, arthralgias, headaches, angina, claudication, erythema nodosum-like lesions; hypertension, bruits, absent pulses, cerebrovascular insufficiency, aortic insufficiency
  - Increased frequency of HLA-Bw52 histocompatibility antigen in Japanese patients, MB3 in North American patients
  - Angiography reveals narrowing, stenosis, and aneurysms of the aortic arch and its major branches
  - Rich collateral flow in the shoulder, chest, and neck areas

- ■ Differential Diagnosis
  - Giant cell arteritis
  - Syphilitic aortitis
  - Severe atherosclerosis

- ■ Treatment
  - Corticosteroids
  - Cyclophosphamide, methotrexate for severe disease
  - Surgical bypass or reconstruction of affected vessels

6

Thromboangiitis Obliterans (Buerger's Disease)

- ■ Essentials of Diagnosis
  - • Inflammatory disease involving small- and medium-sized arteries and veins of the distal extremities
  - • Occurs almost exclusively in young men who are heavy cigarette smokers
  - • Associated with migratory superficial segmental thrombophlebitis of superficial veins, absent peripheral pulses, claudication, numbness, paresthesias, Raynaud's phenomenon, ulceration and gangrene of fingertips and toes
  - • Angiography reveals multiple occluded segments in the small- and medium-sized arteries of the arms and legs

- ■ Differential Diagnosis
  - • Atherosclerosis
  - • Raynaud's phenomenon
  - • Livedo reticularis
  - • Antiphospholipid antibody syndrome
  - • Cholesterol atheroembolic disease

- ■ Treatment
  - • Smoking cessation is essential
  - • Warm clothing, nifedipine for Raynaud's phenomenon
  - • Surgical sympathectomy
  - • Amputation required in some

Behçet's Syndrome

- **Essentials of Diagnosis**
  - Recurrent oral aphthous ulcerations, genital ulcers, ocular lesions (uveitis, hypopyon, iritis, keratitis, optic neuritis), and skin lesions (erythema nodosum, subcutaneous thrombophlebitis, cutaneous hypersensitivity, folliculitis)
  - Usually occurs in young adults; very common in Japan
  - Associated with synovitis, gastrointestinal erosions and ulcers, vasculitis, thrombophlebitis, epididymitis, glomerulonephritis, pulmonary infiltrates, cranial nerve palsies, encephalitis, aseptic meningitis, seizures, spinal cord lesions
  - Diagnosis is clinical
  - HLA-B5 histocompatibility antigen often present

- **Differential Diagnosis**
  - Reactive arthritis
  - Oral aphthous ulcers
  - Herpes simplex infection
  - Erythema multiforme
  - SLE

- **Treatment**
  - Corticosteroids
  - Colchicine
  - Azathioprine, chlorambucil, cyclosporine

6

Ankylosing Spondylitis

■ Essentials of Diagnosis
- Gradual onset of backache in adults under age 40 with progressive limitation of back motion and chest expansion
- Associated with morning back pain and stiffness, chest pain, anterior uveitis, aortic insufficiency, cardiac conduction defects, peripheral arthritis (50%); cauda equina syndrome, apical pulmonary fibrosis are late complications
- Diminished anterior flexion of lumbar spine
- HLA-B27 histocompatibility antigen present in over 90% of patients
- Radiographic evidence of sacroiliac joint sclerosis; demineralization and squaring of the vertebral bodies with calcification of the anterior and lateral spinal ligaments (bamboo spine)

■ Differential Diagnosis
- Rheumatoid arthritis
- Osteoporosis
- Reactive arthritis (Reiter's syndrome)
- Arthritis associated with inflammatory bowel disease
- Psoriatic arthritis
- Diffuse idiopathic skeletal hyperostosis (DISH)

■ Treatment
- Physical therapy to maintain posture and mobility
- NSAIDs (eg, indomethacin 50 mg three times daily)
- Sulfasalazine reported effective in some patients
- Intra-articular corticosteroids for synovitis; ophthalmic corticosteroids for uveitis
- Surgery for severely affected joints

Psoriatic Arthritis

- ■ Essentials of Diagnosis
  - Classically a destructive arthritis of distal interphalangeal joints; many patients also have peripheral oligoarticular disease
  - Occurs in 15–20% of patients with psoriasis
  - Associated with nail pitting, onycholysis, sausage digits, arthritis mutilans (severe deforming arthritis)
  - Sacroiliitis in B27-positive patients
  - Rheumatoid factor negative; uric acid may be elevated
  - Radiographs may reveal irregular destruction of joint spaces and bone, pencil-in-cup deformity of the phalanx, sacroiliitis

- ■ Differential Diagnosis
  - Rheumatoid arthritis
  - Ankylosing spondylitis
  - Arthritis associated with inflammatory bowel disease
  - Reactive arthritis

- ■ Treatment
  - Aspirin (1 g four times daily); other NSAIDs (eg, ibuprofen 800 mg three times daily)
  - Colchicine
  - Intra-articular corticosteroid injection
  - Gold salts, methotrexate
  - Sulfasalazine reported effective in some patients
  - Treatment of psoriasis helpful in many, but not in sacroiliitis

Reactive Arthritis (Reiter's Syndrome)

■ **Essentials of Diagnosis**

- Triad of urethritis, conjunctivitis (or uveitis), and arthritis
- Follows dysenteric infection (with *Shigella, Salmonella, Yersinia, Campylobacter*) or sexually transmitted infection (with *Chlamydia*)
- Asymmetric, oligoarticular arthritis typically involving the knees and ankles
- Associated with fever, mucocutaneous lesions, stomatitis, aortic regurgitation, optic neuritis, balanitis, prostatitis, keratoderma blennorrhagica, pericarditis
- HLA-B27 histocompatibility antigen present in most patients

■ **Differential Diagnosis**

- Gonococcal arthritis
- Rheumatoid arthritis
- Ankylosing spondylitis
- Psoriatic arthritis
- Arthritis associated with inflammatory bowel disease

■ **Treatment**

- NSAIDs (eg, indomethacin, 50 mg three times daily)
- Tetracycline for associated *Chlamydia trachomatis* infection
- Azathioprine, methotrexate in severe cases
- Sulfasalazine reported effective in some patients
- Intra-articular corticosteroids for arthritis, ophthalmic corticosteroids for uveitis

Arthritis Associated With Inflammatory Bowel Disease

- **Essentials of Diagnosis**
  - Two forms of arthritis can occur:
    1. Peripheral arthritis: Asymmetric oligoarthritis that typically involves the knees, ankles, and occasionally the upper extremities and parallels bowel disease in activity
    2. Spondylitis: Clinically identical to ankylosing spondylitis; HLA-B27 antigen present in most patients
  - About 15% of patients will develop arthritis or vasculitis after jejunoileal bypass surgery
  - Articular features may dominate clinical picture or may precede intestinal symptoms

- **Differential Diagnosis**
  - Reactive arthritis
  - Ankylosing spondylitis
  - Psoriatic arthritis
  - Rheumatoid arthritis

- **Treatment**
  - Treat underlying intestinal inflammation
  - Aspirin, other NSAIDs (eg, indomethacin, 50 mg three times daily)
  - Physical therapy for spondylitis

Septic Arthritis (Nongonococcal Acute Bacterial Arthritis)

- ■ Essentials of Diagnosis
  - • Acute pain, swelling, erythema, warmth, and limited movement of joints
  - • Typically monarticular; knee, hip, wrist, shoulder, or ankle most often
  - • Infection usually occurs via hematogenous seeding of the synovium
  - • Previous joint damage or intravenous drug abuse predisposes
  - • Most common organisms: *Staphylococcus aureus,* group A streptococci, *Escherichia coli,* and *Pseudomonas aeruginosa; Haemophilus influenzae* in children under 5; *Staphylococcus epidermidis* following arthroscopy or joint surgery
  - • White cell count in synovial fluid > 100,000/μL; synovial fluid culture positive in 50–75%, blood cultures in 50%

- ■ Differential Diagnosis
  - • Gonococcal arthritis
  - • Gout
  - • Pseudogout
  - • Rheumatoid arthritis
  - • Still's disease
  - • Infective endocarditis
  - • Osteomyelitis

- ■ Treatment
  - • Intravenous antibiotics
  - • Repeated aspiration of affected joint
  - • Rest, immobilization, and elevation
  - • Removal of prosthetic joint

6

Gonococcal Arthritis

- ■ Essentials of Diagnosis
    - Tenosynovitis in many joints followed by monarticular arthritis
    - Characteristic purpuric skin lesions on the distal extremities
    - Most common in young women during menses or pregnancy
    - White cell count in synovial fluid may be up to 100,000/μL; synovial fluid Gram stain positive in 25% of cases; synovial fluid culture positive in less than 50%; blood cultures positive in 40% with tenosynovitis
    - Urethral, throat, and rectal cultures for *Neisseria gonorrhoeae* may be positive in the absence of symptoms
    - Recurrent disseminated gonococcal infection seen with congenital terminal complement component deficiency (C7 and C8)

- ■ Differential Diagnosis
    - Nongonococcal bacterial arthritis
    - Reactive arthritis
    - Lyme disease
    - Sarcoidosis
    - Infective endocarditis

- ■ Treatment
    - Intravenous ceftriaxone or ceftizoxime followed by oral cefixime or ciprofloxacin

Infectious Osteomyelitis

- ■ Essentials of Diagnosis
    - Subacute, vague pain and tenderness of affected bone or back with little or no fever in adults; more acute presentation in children
    - Infection usually occurs via hematogenous seeding of the bone; metaphyses of long bones and vertebrae most frequently involved
    - Organisms include *Staphylococcus aureus,* coagulase-negative staphylococci, group A streptococci, gram-negative rods, anaerobic and polymicrobial infections, tuberculosis, brucellosis, histoplasmosis, coccidioidomycosis, blastomycosis
    - Blood cultures may be positive; aspiration or biopsy of bone is diagnostic
    - Radiographs early in the course are often negative, but periarticular demineralization, erosion of bone, and periostitis may occur later
    - Radionuclide bone scan is 90% sensitive and may be positive within 2 days after onset of symptoms

- ■ Differential Diagnosis
    - Acute bacterial arthritis
    - Rheumatic fever
    - Cellulitis
    - Multiple myeloma
    - Ewing's sarcoma
    - Metastatic neoplasia

- ■ Treatment
    - Intravenous antibiotics after appropriate cultures have been obtained
    - Oral ciprofloxacin, 750 mg twice daily for 6–8 weeks, may be effective
    - Debridement if response to antibiotics is poor

Eosinophilic Fasciitis

- ■ Essentials of Diagnosis
  - Pain, swelling, stiffness, and tenderness of the hands, forearms, feet, or legs evolving to woody induration and retraction of subcutaneous tissue within days to weeks
  - Occurs predominantly in men
  - Associated with peripheral blood eosinophilia, polyarthralgias, arthritis, carpal tunnel syndrome, absence of Raynaud's phenomenon
  - Biopsy of deep fascia is diagnostic
  - Increased risk of aplastic anemia, thrombocytopenia

- ■ Differential Diagnosis
  - Systemic sclerosis
  - Eosinophilia myalgia syndrome
  - Hypothyroidism
  - Trichinosis

- ■ Treatment
  - NSAIDs
  - Short course of corticosteroids

Fibrositis (Fibromyalgia)

- ■ Essentials of Diagnosis
    - Chronic aching pain and stiffness of trunk and extremities, especially around the neck, shoulder, low back, and hips
    - Most frequent in women ages 20–50
    - Associated with multiple tender areas (trigger points), fatigue, headaches, subjective numbness, sleep disorders, irritable bowel symptoms
    - Absence of objective signs of inflammation; normal laboratory studies, including erythrocyte sedimentation rate

- ■ Differential Diagnosis
    - Chronic fatigue syndrome
    - Rheumatoid arthritis
    - SLE
    - Depression
    - Polymyalgia rheumatica

- ■ Treatment
    - Patient education, supportive care, exercise
    - Aspirin, other NSAIDs
    - Tricyclics, benzodiazepines, cyclobenzaprine, chlorpromazine
    - Injection of trigger points with corticosteroids

Amyloidosis

- ### Essentials of Diagnosis
  - A group of disorders characterized by deposition in tissues of ordinarily soluble peptides
  - May be primary (idiopathic or myeloma-associated), familial, localized, or secondary (to familial Mediterranean fever, chronic infectious or inflammatory disease, aging, hemodialysis); in each, a different protein is responsible
  - Associated with peripheral neuropathy, postural hypotension, nephrotic syndrome, cardiomyopathy, arrhythmias, esophageal hypomotility, hepatosplenomegaly, gastrointestinal malabsorption and obstruction, carpal tunnel syndrome, macroglossia, arthropathy, endocrine gland insufficiency, respiratory failure, cutaneous lesions, and ecchymoses
  - Distribution depends on type of amyloid
  - M-spike often seen in primary amyloidosis
  - Amyloid protein (with characteristic green birefringence under polarizing microscope after Congo red staining) may be found on biopsy of rectal mucosa, gingival mucosa, bone marrow, or aspiration of abdominal fat pad in systemic disease

- ### Differential Diagnosis
  - Hemochromatosis
  - Sarcoidosis
  - Waldenström's macroglobulinemia
  - Metastatic neoplasm
  - POEMS syndrome (polyneuropathy, organomegaly, endocrinopathy, M-spike, skin changes)

- ### Treatment
  - Colchicine to prevent attacks of causative familial Mediterranean fever when present
  - Melphalan, prednisone if myeloma-associated
  - Treat underlying disease if present

Reflex Sympathetic Dystrophy

- **Essentials of Diagnosis**
    - Pain and tenderness, most commonly of the hand or foot, associated with vasomotor instability, diffuse swelling, skin atrophy, and hyperhidrosis
    - Usually follows direct trauma to the hand or foot, knee injury, stroke, peripheral nerve injury, or arthroscopic knee surgery
    - Shoulder-hand variant with restricted ipsilateral shoulder movement is common after neck or shoulder injuries or following myocardial infarction
    - Characteristic disparity between severity of the injury and degree of pain
    - Radiographs show severe osteopenia (Sudeck's atrophy); bone scan reveals increased uptake

- **Differential Diagnosis**
    - Rheumatoid arthritis
    - Polymyositis
    - Scleroderma
    - Gout
    - Pseudogout

- **Treatment**
    - Supportive care
    - Physical therapy
    - Active and passive exercises combined with benzodiazepines
    - Stellate ganglion or lumbar sympathetic block
    - Short course of corticosteroids

7

Endocrine Disorders

Panhypopituitarism

- **Essentials of Diagnosis**
  - Sexual dysfunction, weakness, easy fatigability; poor resistance to stress, cold, or fasting; axillary and pubic hair loss
  - Low blood pressure; may have visual field defects
  - Low serum T_4, TSH, GH, FSH, LH, ACTH; low urinary 17-ketosteroids and 17-hydroxycorticosteroids; prolactin level may be elevated
  - CT scan or MRI may reveal sellar lesion

- **Differential Diagnosis**
  - Anorexia nervosa or severe malnutrition
  - Primary adrenal or thyroid disease
  - Cachexia due to other causes (eg, carcinoma or tuberculosis)
  - Empty sella syndrome

- **Treatment**
  - Surgical removal or irradiation of pituitary tumor if present
  - Lifelong endocrine replacement therapy with corticosteroids, thyroid hormone, growth hormone, and sex hormones

Acromegaly & Gigantism

- ■ Essentials of Diagnosis
    - Excessive growth of hands (increased glove size), feet (increased shoe size), jaw (protrusion of lower jaw), face, and tongue; gigantism if prior to epiphysial closure
    - Amenorrhea, headaches, excessive sweating, visual field loss, coarse facial features, deep voice
    - Serum phosphorus > 4 mg/dL, serum T_4 and gonadotropin levels normal or low; hyperglycemia or glycosuria common
    - Elevated insulin-like growth factor (IGF-1)
    - Elevated serum growth hormone with failure of glucose suppression
    - Radiographic findings include sellar enlargement and terminal phalangeal "tufting"; CT or MRI demonstrates pituitary tumor in 90%

- ■ Differential Diagnosis
    - Physiologic growth spurt
    - Familial coarse features
    - Myxedema
    - Pachydermoperiostosis

- ■ Treatment
    - Most patients have a partial response to somatostatin analogs (eg, octreotide)
    - Bromocriptine may control growth hormone secretion
    - Transsphenoidal resection of adenoma is successful in most patients; pituitary irradiation may be necessary if surgery fails
    - Residual panhypopituitarism may require hormonal replacement ("burnout" acromegaly)

Hyperprolactinemia

- ■ Essentials of Diagnosis
  - Women: menstrual disturbance (oligomenorrhea, amenorrhea); galactorrhea, infertility
  - Men: erectile dysfunction and decreased libido, hypogonadism; galactorrhea, infertility
  - Serum prolactin usually > 100 ng/mL
  - May be caused by hypothyroidism
  - Pituitary adenoma often demonstrated by CT or MRI

- ■ Differential Diagnosis
  - Hypothyroidism
  - Pregnancy or other causes of amenorrhea
  - Other causes of male impotence or hypogonadism
  - Use of prolactin-stimulating drugs

- ■ Treatment
  - Dopamine agonists (eg, bromocriptine or pergolide) usually shrink pituitary adenoma and restore fertility
  - Transsphenoidal resection for large tumors, those causing visual compromise or refractory to dopamine agonists

7

Diabetes Insipidus

- ■ Essentials of Diagnosis
  - Polydipsia and polyuria to volumes of 2–20 L/d; intensive thirst
  - Urine specific gravity < 1.006; random serum osmolality > 290 mosm/L
  - Inability to concentrate urine with fluid restriction
  - Classified into primary diabetes insipidus, secondary diabetes insipidus (due to damage to the hypothalamus or pituitary stalk by trauma, anoxia, or infection), pregnancy-associated diabetes insipidus, and nephrogenic diabetes insipidus
  - Vasopressin challenge reduces urine output (except in nephrogenic diabetes insipidus)

- ■ Differential Diagnosis
  - Psychogenic polydipsia
  - Central nervous system sarcoidosis
  - Diabetes mellitus
  - Hypercalcemia
  - Hyperkalemia

- ■ Treatment
  - Intranasal desmopressin acetate once or twice daily
  - Ensure adequate fluid intake in all cases
  - Chlorpropamide also effective for partial diabetes insipidus (non-nephrogenic)
  - Hydrochlorothiazide, indomethacin, or amiloride for nephrogenic diabetes insipidus

Simple & Nodular Goiter

- ■ Essentials of Diagnosis
  - Symptoms are associated with compression of surrounding structures by large thyroid gland (dysphagia, respiratory difficulty)
  - Enlarged, often nodular thyroid gland palpable
  - T_4 normal; TSH may be normal or elevated; radioactive iodine uptake normal or elevated

- ■ Differential Diagnosis
  - Toxic goiter
  - Autoimmune thyroiditis
  - Carcinoma of the thyroid

- ■ Treatment
  - Levothyroxine replacement to suppress TSH
  - Iodine only if goiter related to deficiency
  - Surgery for severe local symptoms or if malignancy cannot be excluded; fine-needle aspiration of single cold nodules used to exclude malignancy

7

Adult Hypothyroidism & Myxedema

- ## Essentials of Diagnosis
  - Weakness, fatigue, cold intolerance, constipation, menstrual disturbance, hoarse voice, altered mentation, depression, weight gain or loss, deafness
  - Bradycardia; dry, cold, yellow, puffy skin; thin eyebrows; macroglossia; delayed return of deep tendon reflexes
  - Serum T_4 < 3.5 mg/dL, free T_4 < 0.8 mg/dL; radioiodine uptake < 10%/24 hours; TSH elevated in primary myxedema

- ## Differential Diagnosis
  - Chronic fatigue
  - Malnutrition
  - Congestive heart failure
  - Primary amyloidosis
  - Depression

- ## Treatment
  - Levothyroxine replacement starting with low doses and increasing gradually
  - Treat myxedema coma (a medical emergency) with intravenous levothyroxine and hydrocortisone

Hyperthyroidism

- ■ Essentials of Diagnosis
  - Nervousness, weight loss with increased appetite, heat intolerance, weakness, increased bowel frequency, polyuria, menstrual disturbances, infertility
  - Sinus tachycardia or atrial fibrillation, warm moist skin, goiter, thyroid thrill or bruit, gynecomastia, proximal weakness, eye findings (stare, lid lag, exophthalmos)
  - Serum T_4 and radioiodine T_3 resin uptake both increased; TSH low to absent; lymphocytosis, hypocalcemia, glycosuria common
  - Thyroid-stimulating immunoglobulin, antithyroid antibody often positive in Graves' disease

- ■ Differential Diagnosis
  - Anxiety, neurosis, or mania
  - Pheochromocytoma
  - Malignancy
  - Chronic alcoholism
  - Primary myopathy
  - Myasthenia gravis
  - Exogenous thyroid administration

- ■ Treatment
  - Methimazole or propylthiouracil for patients with mild thyrotoxicosis or small goiters
  - Propranolol for symptomatic relief of catecholamine-mediated symptoms
  - Radioactive iodine for severe or refractory cases (contraindicated in pregnancy)
  - Subtotal thyroidectomy for failure of medical therapy or for large goiters; euthyroid state must be achieved medically prior to surgery

Thyroiditis

- **Essentials of Diagnosis**
    - Painful swelling of thyroid gland with local pressure symptoms and referred ear pain in acute and subacute forms; painless enlargement in chronic form
    - Painful, enlarged thyroid; symptoms of hyperthyroidism variable
    - Classified as chronic lymphocytic (Hashimoto's) thyroiditis, subacute thyroiditis, suppurative thyroiditis, or Riedel's thyroiditis
    - Thyroid function tests variable, with serum T_4 and T_3 levels often high in acute forms and reduced in chronic disease; leukocytosis, elevated erythrocyte sedimentation rate, and elevated serum globulins common
    - Radioiodine uptake uniformly reduced
    - Thyroid autoantibodies positive in Hashimoto's thyroiditis

- **Differential Diagnosis**
    - Endemic goiter
    - Hyperthyroidism due to other causes
    - Carcinoma of the thyroid
    - Pyogenic infections of the neck

- **Treatment**
    - Antibiotics for suppurative thyroiditis
    - Aspirin for subacute thyroiditis; prednisone in severe cases
    - Symptomatic treatment with propranolol
    - Levothyroxine for Hashimoto's thyroiditis
    - Partial thyroidectomy for local severe pressure or adhesions in Riedel's thyroiditis

7

Hypoparathyroidism

- **Essentials of Diagnosis**
  - History of previous thyroidectomy or neck surgery present in most patients
  - Tetany, carpopedal spasms, stridor or wheezing, tingling distal limbs and lips, muscle or abdominal cramps, urinary frequency, altered mentation
  - Positive Chvostek sign (facial muscle contraction on tapping the facial nerve) and Trousseau phenomenon (carpal spasm after application of a cuff); defective nails and teeth; cataracts
  - Serum calcium low; serum phosphate high; urinary phosphate low, urine calcium low; serum parathyroid hormone low to absent
  - Alkaline phosphatase normal in hypoparathyroidism but elevated in pseudohypoparathyroidism
  - Basal ganglia calcification may be seen by radiograph or CT scan

- **Differential Diagnosis**
  - Tetany due to respiratory alkalosis
  - Vitamin D deficiency syndromes
  - Acute pancreatitis
  - Hypomagnesemia
  - Chronic renal failure
  - Epilepsy or structural disease of the brain

- **Treatment**
  - For acute tetany, intravenous calcium gluconate, followed by oral calcium carbonate and vitamin D derivatives
  - Correct concurrent hypomagnesemia
  - Chronic therapy includes high-calcium diet in addition to calcium and vitamin D supplements
  - Avoid phenothiazines (prolonged QT) and furosemide (enhances hypocalcemia)

Primary Hyperparathyroidism

■ **Essentials of Diagnosis**

- Renal stones, bone pain, mental status changes, constipation, polyuria, hypertension; most patients asymptomatic however
- History of renal stones, nephrocalcinosis, hypertension, recurrent peptic ulcer disease, or recurrent pancreatitis often present
- Hypertension, kyphosis, band keratopathy, clubbing on occasion
- Serum and urine calcium elevated; urine phosphate high with low or normal serum phosphate; alkaline phosphatase elevated if bone disease present
- Elevated parathyroid hormone levels confirm diagnosis
- Bone radiographs show subperiosteal resorption of phalanges, dental loss of lamina dura, nephrocalcinosis or nephrolithiasis, bone cysts or pathologic fractures ("osteitis fibrosa"), chondrocalcinosis; many adenomas visible on ultrasonography

■ **Differential Diagnosis**

- Vitamin D intoxication
- Sarcoidosis or other granulomatous disorders
- Hyperthyroidism
- Multiple myeloma
- Milk-alkali syndrome
- Hypercalcemia of malignancy
- Thiazide therapy
- Adrenal insufficiency
- Familial hypocalciuric hypercalcemia

■ **Treatment**

- Parathyroidectomy for patients with symptomatic hyperparathyroidism, kidney stones, or bone disease
- Bisphosphonates (eg, pamidronate) for acute treatment of severe hypercalcemia while preparing for surgery
- For asymptomatic patients: maintain adequate fluid intake and avoid immobilization, thiazide diuretics, and calcium-containing antacids
- Estrogen replacement for postmenopausal women

7

Osteoporosis

■ **Essentials of Diagnosis**
  • Asymptomatic or associated with back pain, spontaneous fractures, loss of height
  • Kyphosis, spinal tenderness
  • Serum calcium, phosphorus, parathyroid hormone, and alkaline phosphatase levels normal
  • Demineralization of spine, hip, and pelvis by radiograph, vertebral compression fractures

■ **Differential Diagnosis**
  • Osteomalacia
  • Hyperparathyroidism
  • Multiple myeloma
  • Metastatic carcinoma
  • Hypophosphatasia
  • Osteogenesis imperfecta

■ **Treatment**
  • Estrogens to decrease bone resorption in postmenopausal women
  • Diet adequate in protein, calcium, and vitamin D plus supplemental calcium carbonate and vitamin D
  • Calcitonin
  • Regular exercise
  • Thiazides if hypercalciuria present

Polyostotic Fibrous Dysplasia

- ■ Essentials of Diagnosis
  - Painless swelling of involved bones; fractures with minimal trauma; begins in childhood
  - Brown pigmentation sometimes present in skin overlying bony lesions
  - Bone cysts or hyperostotic lesions, usually multiple, in segmental distribution by x-ray
  - Variety of endocrinopathies may be associated ("McCune-Albright syndrome")

- ■ Differential Diagnosis
  - Hyperparathyroidism
  - Neurofibromatosis
  - Paget's disease
  - Other bone cysts and tumors

- ■ Treatment
  - Surgical correction of fractures and deformities

Paget's Disease (Osteitis Deformans)

- ■ Essentials of Diagnosis
  - Asymptomatic or associated with bone pain and frequent fractures with minimal trauma
  - Kyphosis, bowed tibias, large head, warmth over involved bones
  - Alkaline phosphatase and urinary hydroxyproline markedly elevated; serum calcium and phosphate normal
  - Radiographically dense, expanded bones with destructive cystic lesions in the skull ("osteoporosis circumscripta")

- ■ Differential Diagnosis
  - Osteogenic sarcoma
  - Multiple myeloma
  - Fibrous dysplasia
  - Hyperparathyroidism
  - Metastatic carcinoma
  - Osteitis fibrosis cystica

- ■ Treatment
  - No treatment for asymptomatic patients
  - Calcitonins may be used to reduce osteoclastic activity
  - Bisphosphonates (eg, pamidronate) may be used to inhibit osteoclast-mediated bone resorption

7

Osteomalacia & Rickets

- **Essentials of Diagnosis**
  - Painful proximal muscle weakness, listlessness, aching and "bowing" of bones
  - Defective mineralization of the growing skeleton causes permanent bone deformities in children (rickets) or decreased bone density in adults (osteomalacia)
  - Serum and urine calcium low to normal; serum phosphate low; elevated alkaline phosphatase; decreased 25-hydroxyvitamin D; secondary hyperparathyroidism
  - "Pseudofractures" and "washed out" bone on x-ray
  - Caused by any condition that results in inadequate calcium or phosphate mineralization of bone osteoid (eg, malabsorption, vitamin D deficiency, calcium deficiency, phosphate deficiency)

- **Differential Diagnosis**
  - Osteogenesis imperfecta (children)
  - Osteoporosis (may coexist)
  - Chronic alcoholism
  - Hyperparathyroidism
  - Hypoparathyroidism

- **Treatment**
  - Treatment of underlying disorder
  - Ergocalciferol for vitamin D deficiency
  - Calcifediol or calcitriol for vitamin D resistance syndromes
  - Phosphate supplementation for phosphate deficiency
  - Oral calcium for nutritional calcium deficiency

7

Acute Adrenal Insufficiency

- **Essentials of Diagnosis**
  - Weakness, fever, nausea and vomiting, abdominal pain, confusion
  - Hypotension, dehydration; increased skin pigmentation may be seen
  - Serum potassium high with low serum sodium; lymphocytosis, eosinophilia, azotemia, hypoglycemia, and hypercalcemia often present
  - Serum cortisol does not increase appropriately following administration of cosyntropin (ACTH)
  - Associated with stress, including trauma, surgery, infection, pituitary necrosis, adrenal hemorrhage, or exogenous corticosteroid withdrawal

- **Differential Diagnosis**
  - Bacterial sepsis
  - Hyponatremia from other causes (SIADH, cirrhosis, congestive heart failure)
  - Salt-wasting nephropathy
  - Acute abdomen from other causes
  - Cerebrovascular accident
  - Poisoning
  - Metabolic encephalopathy, eg, diabetic coma

- **Treatment**
  - Immediate intravenous hydrocortisone (100–300 mg intravenously) once the diagnosis is suspected
  - Appropriate volume resuscitation and pressor support for blood pressure
  - Broad-spectrum antibiotics pending exclusion of septicemia
  - Identify and treat precipitating cause

Chronic Adrenocortical Insufficiency (Addison's Disease)

- ■ Essentials of Diagnosis
  - Weakness, easy fatigability, anorexia, weight loss, nausea, vomiting, diarrhea, abdominal pain, myalgias, arthralgias, amenorrhea
  - Hypotension; sparse axillary and pubic hair; increased skin pigmentation at creases, pressure areas, and nipples
  - Low serum sodium and chloride; serum potassium or calcium may be elevated; azotemia, neutropenia, anemia, eosinophilia, and relative lymphocytosis may be present
  - Plasma cortisol levels low to absent and fail to rise after cosyntropin (ACTH) stimulation
  - Plasma ACTH level elevated

- ■ Differential Diagnosis
  - Anorexia nervosa
  - Malabsorption states
  - Occult malignancy
  - Hyperparathyroidism
  - Thyrotoxicosis
  - Panhypopituitarism
  - Hemochromatosis

- ■ Treatment
  - Replacement therapy, including glucocorticoids (hydrocortisone) and mineralocorticoids (fludrocortisone)
  - Increased glucocorticoid supplementation for trauma, surgery, infection, or stress

7

Hypercortisolism (Cushing's Syndrome)

- ■ Essentials of Diagnosis
  - Weakness, muscle wasting, weight gain, hirsutism, menstrual disturbance, thin skin, easy bruisability, psychologic changes, acne, headache
  - Hypertension, centripetal obesity with "moon facies" and "buffalo hump," purple striae, poor wound healing
  - Hyperglycemia, glycosuria, hypokalemia, leukocytosis, lymphocytopenia
  - Elevated serum cortisol and urinary free cortisol; failure of suppression of cortisol secretion by exogenous dexamethasone
  - Osteoporosis common; CT or MRI may reveal adrenal tumor if present

- ■ Differential Diagnosis
  - Chronic alcoholism
  - Depression
  - Diabetes mellitus
  - Adrenogenital syndrome (may be associated)
  - Idiopathic hirsutism
  - Exogenous steroid administration
  - Osteoporosis from other causes
  - Severe obesity

- ■ Treatment
  - Transsphenoidal resection or irradiation of pituitary adenoma if present
  - Resection of adrenal or extra-adrenal tumor if present
  - Bilateral adrenalectomy for adrenal hyperplasia
  - Ketoconazole or metyrapone to suppress cortisol in unresectable adrenal carcinoma

7

Hirsutism & Virilizing Diseases of Women

- ■ Essentials of Diagnosis
  - Menstrual disorders, hirsutism, odorous perspiration, balding, hoarse voice, acne, increased muscularity
  - Occasionally palpable pelvic mass, enlargement of clitoris
  - 17-Ketosteroids and serum DHEAS and androstenedione elevated in adrenal disorders
  - Serum testosterone often elevated
  - Hirsutism may be idiopathic or secondary to polycystic ovary syndrome, adrenal enzyme defects, congenital adrenal hyperplasia, ovarian tumors, adrenal carcinoma, acromegaly, ACTH-induced Cushing's syndrome, or drugs.

- ■ Differential Diagnosis
  - Familial, racial, or idiopathic hirsutism
  - Cushing's syndrome
  - Exogenous androgen ingestion

- ■ Treatment
  - Surgical removal of ovarian or adrenal tumor if present
  - Oral contraceptives to ameliorate hirsutism and normalize menses
  - Spironolactone, finasteride, flutamide, or leuprolide may be used to suppress serum androgens

7

Male Hypogonadism

- **Essentials of Diagnosis**
  - Diminished libido and poor erections
  - Sparse growth of body hair
  - Testes may be small or normal in size; serum testosterone is usually decreased
  - Serum gonadotropins (LH and FSH) are decreased in hypogonadotropic hypogonadism; they are increased in testicular failure (hypergonadotropic hypogonadism)
  - Causes of hypogonadotropic hypogonadism with low or normal LH include chronic illness, malnourishment, hypothyroidism, drugs, Cushing's syndrome, and congenital syndromes
  - Causes of hypergonadotropic hypogonadism with high LH include Klinefelter's syndrome, bilateral anorchia, testicular trauma, orchitis, and myotonic dystrophy

- **Differential Diagnosis**
  - Cushing's syndrome
  - Hemochromatosis
  - Pituitary tumor

- **Treatment**
  - Testosterone intramuscularly

7

Primary Hyperaldosteronism

- ■ Essentials of Diagnosis
  - Muscular weakness, paresthesias and tetany, polyuria, polydipsia, moderate hypertension, headache
  - Hypokalemia, hypernatremia, alkalosis
  - Elevated urine and plasma aldosterone levels with low plasma renin level
  - May be associated with adrenocortical adenoma or bilateral cortical hyperplasia
  - Adrenal mass often demonstrated by CT or MRI

- ■ Differential Diagnosis
  - Essential hypertension
  - Periodic paralysis
  - Hypokalemia due to other causes
  - Excessive ingestion of English licorice, diuretics, or laxatives
  - Unilateral renovascular disease
  - Nephrogenic diabetes insipidus
  - Salt-wasting nephropathies

- ■ Treatment
  - Surgical resection of unilateral adenoma secreting aldosterone
  - Spironolactone for bilateral adrenal hyperplasia
  - Dexamethasone may be used for suppression of hyperplasia
  - Bilateral adrenalectomy corrects the hypokalemia but not the hypertension and should not be performed
  - Antihypertensive therapy as necessary

Pheochromocytoma

- ■ Essentials of Diagnosis
  - Episodes of headaches, palpitations, visual blurring, nausea, sweats, dyspnea, anxiety, tremor, or vasomotor changes; weight loss
  - Hypertension, paroxysmal or sustained; postural tachycardia and hypotension; cardiomegaly; pallor
  - Hypermetabolism with normal thyroid tests; hyperglycemia and glycosuria may be present
  - Elevated urinary catecholamines, metanephrines, and vanillyl-mandelic acid (VMA) are diagnostic; serum epinephrine and nor-epinephrine elevated
  - CT or MRI can confirm and localize pheochromocytoma; ^{123}I MIBG scan may help to localize tumors

- ■ Differential Diagnosis
  - Essential hypertension
  - Other causes of secondary hypertension
  - Thyrotoxicosis
  - Myocarditis
  - Glomerulonephritis
  - Preeclampsia-eclampsia
  - Psychoneurosis
  - Acute intermittent porphyria

- ■ Treatment
  - Surgical removal of tumor or tumors
  - First alpha- then beta-adrenergic receptor blockade and adequate volume replenishment mandatory prior to surgery
  - Oral phenoxybenzamine or metyrosine for symptomatic treatment in patients with inoperable tumors

7

Hypoglycemia in the Adult

- **Essentials of Diagnosis**
  - Blurred vision, diplopia, headache, slurred speech, weakness, sweating, palpitations, tremulousness, altered mentation
  - Plasma glucose < 40 mg/dL
  - Causes include alcoholism, postprandial (eg, postgastrectomy), anti-insulin antibodies or antibodies to insulin receptors, pancreatic B cell tumor, extrapancreatic tumors, adrenal or pituitary insufficiency, medications (sulfonylureas, pentamidine, streptozocin), exogenous insulin use

- **Differential Diagnosis**
  - Central nervous system disease
  - Hypoxia
  - Psychoneurosis
  - Pheochromocytoma

- **Treatment**
  - Intravenous glucose
  - Intramuscular glucagon if no intravenous access available
  - Treatment of underlying disease or removal of offending agent (eg, alcohol, pentamidine)

Type I Diabetes Mellitus (IDDM = Insulin-Dependent Diabetes Mellitus)

- ■ Essentials of Diagnosis
  - Rapid onset polyuria, polydipsia, polyphagia, weight loss, nocturnal enuresis
  - Fasting serum glucose > 140 mg/dL; ketosis common; glycosuria and ketonuria; elevated glycosylated hemoglobin
  - May present as medical emergency (diabetic ketoacidosis); patients are at risk for chronic multiple system dysfunction (eg, cardiovascular disease, renal disease, ocular disease, neuropathy)

- ■ Differential Diagnosis
  - Glycosuria with low renal resorptive threshold
  - Diabetes insipidus
  - Hormonal tumors
  - Medications (eg, glucocorticoids, thiazides, phenytoin)
  - Acanthosis nigricans syndromes

- ■ Treatment
  - Insulin required by definition
  - Patient education is crucial, emphasizing dietary management, exercise, weight loss, foot and eye care
  - Frequent medical visits and follow-ups and home blood sugar determinations important

7

Type II Diabetes Mellitus (NIDDM = Non-Insulin-Dependent Diabetes Mellitus)

■ **Essentials of Diagnosis**

- Most patients are over 40 years of age and obese
- Gradual onset of polyuria, polydipsia; often asymptomatic
- Candidal vaginitis in women, chronic skin infection, generalized pruritus, blurred vision
- Fasting serum glucose > 140 mg/dL on two separate occasions; glycosuria, elevated glycosylated hemoglobin; ketosis rare
- Family history often present; hypertension, hyperlipidemia, and atherosclerosis often associated
- May present as medical emergency (especially in elderly) as nonketotic hyperosmolar coma; patients at risk as in type I diabetes for chronic multisystem disease

■ **Differential Diagnosis**

- Glycosuria with low renal resorptive threshold
- Diabetes insipidus
- Hormonal tumors
- Medications (eg, glucocorticoids, thiazides, phenytoin)
- Acanthosis nigricans syndromes

■ **Treatment**

- Patient education is important, emphasizing dietary management, exercise, weight loss, foot and eye care
- Patients may be controlled with diet, exercise, and weight loss alone
- Oral hypoglycemics if diet ineffective
- Insulin may be required for glycemic control if refractory to diet and oral agents

Diabetic Ketoacidosis

- ■ Essentials of Diagnosis
  - Acute polyuria and polydipsia, marked fatigue, nausea and vomiting, coma
  - "Fruity" breath, hypotension and dehydration, Kussmaul respirations
  - Hyperglycemia > 250 mg/dL, ketonemia, acidemia with blood pH < 7.3 and serum bicarbonate < 15 meq/L, elevated anion gap; glycosuria and ketonuria; total body potassium depleted despite elevation in serum potassium
  - Multiple inciting stressors associated, including myocardial ischemia, surgery, infection, gastroenteritis, intra-abdominal disease, medical noncompliance

- ■ Differential Diagnosis
  - Alcoholic ketoacidosis
  - Uremia
  - Cerebral vascular accidents or head trauma
  - Lactic acidosis
  - Sepsis

- ■ Treatment
  - Aggressive volume resuscitation with saline; dextrose should be added to intravenous fluids once glucose reaches 250–300 mg/dL
  - Intravenous regular insulin replacement with frequent laboratory monitoring
  - Potassium, magnesium, and phosphate replacement
  - Identify and treat inciting stressor

Hyperosmotic Nonketotic Diabetic Coma

- ■ Essentials of Diagnosis
    - • Insidious onset of weakness, polyuria and polydipsia, and dehydration progressing to obtundation, seizure, and coma
    - • Sign of dehydration on physical examination, Kussmaul respirations, lethargy
    - • Profound hyperglycemia (> 600 mg/dL), hypernatremia, hyperosmolality (> 310 mosm/kg); prerenal azotemia; ketosis and acidemia usually absent
    - • Chronically reduced intake of fluids (eg, inability to sense or regulate thirst, or inaccessibility of fluids to elderly) is common setting

- ■ Differential Diagnosis
    - • Cerebral vascular accident or head trauma
    - • Diabetes insipidus

- ■ Treatment
    - • Aggressive volume resuscitation with normal saline until patient euvolemic, then with hypotonic saline
    - • Regular insulin 15 units intravenously plus 15 units subcutaneously initially, then subcutaneously every 4 hours
    - • Careful monitoring of serum sodium, osmolality, and glucose
    - • Dextrose-containing fluids when glucose is 250–300 mg/dL
    - • Potassium and phosphate replacement

7

8

Infectious Diseases

VIRAL INFECTIONS

Herpes Simplex

- **Essentials of Diagnosis**
  - Recurrent grouped small vesicles on erythematous base, usually perioral or perigenital
  - Primary infection associated with fever, regional lymphadenopathy, and malaise
  - Recurrences often precipitated by minor infections, trauma, stress, sun exposure
  - Genital lesions highly infectious through venereal contact
  - Systemic infection with encephalitis may occur in immunosuppressed patients
  - Proctitis, esophagitis, and keratitis may complicate
  - Tzanck smear or ulcer scraping positive for large multinucleated epithelial cells

- **Differential Diagnosis**
  - Herpangina
  - Aphthous ulcers
  - Stevens-Johnson syndrome
  - Bacterial infection of the skin
  - Syphilis and other sexually transmitted diseases
  - Other causes of encephalitis, proctitis, or keratitis

- **Treatment**
  - Acyclovir may attenuate recurrent course of genital or oral lesion and should be given for systemic or central nervous system disease

Measles (Rubeola)

- ■ Essentials of Diagnosis
    - An acute systemic viral illness transmitted by inhalation of infective droplets
    - Incubation period 10–14 days
    - Prodrome of fever, coryza, cough, conjunctivitis, photophobia
    - Onset of brick-red, irregular maculopapular rash 3 days after prodrome from face to trunk to extremities
    - Koplik's spots (tiny "table salt crystals") on the buccal mucosa are pathognomonic, but occur and disappear rapidly
    - Leukopenia
    - Encephalitis in 1–3%

- ■ Differential Diagnosis
    - Other acute exanthems (eg, rubella, enterovirus, Epstein-Barr virus infection, varicella, roseola)
    - Drug allergy

- ■ Treatment
    - Primary immunization preventive after age 15 months; revaccination of adults born after 1957 without documented immunity recommended
    - Isolation for 1 week following onset of rash
    - Specific treatment of secondary bacterial complications

8

Rubella *German Measles*

"3 Day"

■ **Essentials of Diagnosis**

- A systemic viral illness transmitted by inhalation of infected droplets
- Incubation period 14–21 days
- No prodrome in children (mild in adults); fever, malaise, coryza coincide with eruption of fine maculopapular rash on face to trunk to extremities which rapidly fades
- Arthralgias common, particularly in young women
- Posterior cervical, suboccipital, and posterior auricular lymphadenopathy 5–10 days before rash
- Leukopenia, thrombocytopenia
- In one out of 6000 cases, postinfectious encephalopathy develops 1–6 days after the rash; mortality rate is 20%

■ **Differential Diagnosis**

- Other acute exanthems (eg, rubeola, enterovirus, Epstein-Barr virus infection, varicella)

■ **Treatment**

- Active immunization after age 15 months; girls should be immunized before menarche though not during pregnancy
- Symptomatic therapy only

CRS - Congenital Rubella Syndrome

Cytomegalovirus Disease

- ■ Essentials of Diagnosis
  - Neonatal infection; hepatosplenomegaly, purpura, central nervous system abnormalities
  - Immunocompetent adults: malaise, fever, myalgias, hepatosplenomegaly, leukopenia with lymphocytic predominance, often following transfusion
  - Immunocompromised adults: pneumonia, meningoencephalitis, chorioretinitis, chronic diarrhea
  - Fever may be prolonged
  - Viral cultures of affected tissues diagnostic, IgM antibody rise, urinary cytologic examination also of value

- ■ Differential Diagnosis
  - Infectious mononucleosis (Epstein-Barr virus)
  - Other causes of prolonged fever (eg, lymphoma, endocarditis)
  - In immunocompromised patients: other causes of atypical pneumonia, meningoencephalitis, or chronic diarrhea
  - In infants: toxoplasmosis, rubella, herpes simplex, syphilis

- ■ Treatment
  - Appropriate supportive care
  - Ganciclovir or foscarnet intravenously

Varicella (Acute Chickenpox, Zoster [Shingles])

- ■ Essentials of Diagnosis
  - Acute varicella: fever, malaise with eruption of pruritic, centripetal, papular rash, vesicular and pustular before crusting—lesions in all stages at any given time
  - Incubation period 14–21 days
  - Bacterial infection, pneumonia, and encephalitis may complicate
  - Reactivation varicella (herpes zoster): dermatomal distribution, vesicular rash with pain often preceding eruption

- ■ Differential Diagnosis
  - Other viral infections
  - Drug allergy

lesions on nose—nasociliary branch of CN V,

- ■ Treatment
  - Supportive measures with topical lotions and antihistamines
  - Immune globulin for exposed susceptible immunosuppressed patients
  - Acyclovir early for immunocompromised patients, severe disease (pneumonitis), or ophthalmic division of trigeminal nerve involvement with zoster
  - Corticosteroids with rapid taper may diminish postherpetic neuralgia in elderly patients with zoster

8

Mumps (Epidemic Parotitis)

■ Essentials of Diagnosis
  • Painful, swollen salivary glands (may be unilateral), usually parotid; fever, sore throat
  • Orchitis or oophoritis, meningoencephalitis, or pancreatitis may occur
  • Cerebrospinal fluid shows lymphocytic pleocytosis in meningoencephalitis with hypoglycorrhachia
  • Incubation period 12–24 days
  • Diagnosis confirmed by isolation of virus in saliva or appearance of antibodies after second week

■ Differential Diagnosis
  • Parotitis due to other causes (eg, bacteria, calculi, Sjögren's syndrome, sarcoidosis, parotid malignancy)
  • Aseptic meningitis, pancreatitis, epididymitis, or orchitis due to other causes

■ Treatment
  • Immunization is preventive
  • Supportive care with surveillance for complications

Viral Encephalitis

- ■ Essentials of Diagnosis
  - Agents include arbovirus, herpes simplex, enterovirus, measles, rubella, rubeola, varicella, Epstein-Barr virus
  - Fever, malaise, stiff neck, sore throat, nausea, altered mentation
  - Signs of upper motor neuron lesion: exaggerated deep tendon reflexes, absent superficial reflexes, spastic paralysis
  - Cerebrospinal fluid protein and pressure often increased with lymphocytic pleocytosis
  - Isolation of virus from blood or cerebrospinal fluid; serology positive in paired specimens 3–4 weeks apart
  - MRI of the brain abnormal in the temporal lobes in herpetic encephalitis

- ■ Differential Diagnosis
  - Other encephalitides (post vaccination, Reye's syndrome, toxins)
  - Aseptic meningitis
  - Lymphocytic choriomeningitis
  - Nonparalytic poliomyelitis
  - Primary or secondary neoplasm
  - Purulent meningitis or brain abscess

- ■ Treatment
  - Vigorous supportive measures with attention to elevated central nervous system pressures
  - Corticosteroids, mannitol in selected patients
  - Acyclovir for herpes simplex encephalitis; otherwise no specific antiviral therapy available

Poliomyelitis

- ■ Essentials of Diagnosis
  - Acquired via fecal-oral route
  - Muscle weakness, malaise, headache, fever, nausea, abdominal pain, sore throat
  - Signs of lower motor neuron lesions: asymmetric, flaccid paralysis with decreased deep tendon reflexes, muscle atrophy; may include cranial nerve abnormalities (bulbar form)
  - Cerebrospinal fluid lymphocytic pleocytosis with slight elevation of protein
  - Virus recovered from throat washings or stool

- ■ Differential Diagnosis
  - Other aseptic meningitides
  - Postinfectious polyneuropathy (Guillain-Barré syndrome)

- ■ Treatment
  - Vaccination is preventive
  - Supportive care with particular attention to respiratory function, skin care, and bowel and bladder function

8

Lymphocytic Choriomeningitis

- ### Essentials of Diagnosis
  - History of exposure to mice or hamsters
  - "Influenza-like" prodrome with fever, chills, headache, malaise, and cough followed by headache, photophobia, or neck pain
  - Kernig and Brudzinski signs positive
  - Cerebrospinal fluid with lymphocytic pleocytosis and slight increase in protein
  - Serology for arenavirus positive 2 weeks after onset of symptoms
  - Virus recovered from blood and cerebrospinal fluid
  - The illness usually lasts 1–2 weeks

- ### Differential Diagnosis
  - Other aseptic meningitides
  - Bacterial or granulomatous meningitis

- ### Treatment
  - Supportive care

8

Dengue (Breakbone Fever, Dandy Fever)

- **Essentials of Diagnosis**
    - A viral (togavirus, flavivirus) illness transmitted by the bite of the *Aedes* mosquito
    - Sudden onset of high fever, chills, severe aching, headache, sore throat
    - Biphasic fever curve with initial phase of 3–4 days, a short remission, and a second phase of 1–2 days
    - Rash is maculopapular, scarlatiniform, morbilliform, or petechial and occurs during remission or second phase of fever, beginning in the extremities and spreading to the torso
    - Dengue hemorrhagic fever is a severe form in which gastrointestinal hemorrhage is prominent and patients often present with shock

- **Differential Diagnosis**
    - Malaria
    - Yellow fever
    - Influenza
    - Typhoid fever
    - Meningococcemia
    - Sepsis
    - Toxic shock syndrome
    - Rickettsial disease
    - Other viral exanthems

- **Treatment**
    - Supportive care
    - Effective vaccine available but not commercially available

HIV Infection (AIDS)

- **Essentials of Diagnosis**
  - Caused by a retrovirus slowly destroying CD4 lymphocytes
  - At risk populations include intravenous drug users, blood product recipients, health care workers injured with needles used for HIV-positive patients, homosexual men; heterosexual transmission common in much of the world
  - Acute HIV infection characterized by nonspecific flu-like syndrome and aseptic meningitis
  - Later, opportunistic infections, certain malignancies and AIDS wasting dictate the clinical picture, two to 15 years after primary infection
  - Picture deteriorates as CD4 count falls below 200

- **Differential Diagnosis**
  - Depends upon which infection is complicating
  - Interstitial lung diseases of numerous types
  - Non-AIDS lymphoma
  - Tuberculosis
  - Sarcoidosis
  - Brain abscess
  - FUO of other cause
  - Posterior uveitis of other causes

- **Treatment**
  - Antiretrovirals and protease inhibitors in combination now shown to prolong life   *p. 281*
  - Prophylaxis for pneumocystis when CD4 count reaches 200
  - Otherwise, treatment for associated lymphoma, toxoplasmosis, mycobacteriosis, CMV, Kaposi's as indicated

PCP prophy
TMP/SMX
dapsone
Atovaquone
Pentamidine

MAI prophy
Zithromax

Toxo prophy
SMX or
Pyramethamine

Rabies

- **Essentials of Diagnosis**
  - A rhabdovirus encephalitis transmitted by infected saliva
  - History of animal bite (bears, skunks, foxes, raccoons, and dogs and cats in developing countries)
  - Paresthesias, hydrophobia, rage alternating with calm
  - Convulsions, paralysis, thick tenacious saliva, and muscle spasms

- **Differential Diagnosis**
  - Tetanus
  - Encephalitis due to other causes

- **Treatment**
  - Active immunization of household pets and persons at risk (eg, veterinarians)
  - Thorough, repeated washing of bite and scratch wounds
  - Postexposure immunization, both passive and active
  - Observation of healthy biting animals, examination of brains of sick or dead biting animals
  - Treatment is supportive only; the disease is almost uniformly fatal

PEP → Vaccine (Ag) (0,3,7,14,28°)

Immunization (Ab)
RIG (.133 mg/kg)
50% im/around wound if possible

Yellow Fever

- ## Essentials of Diagnosis
    - Arbovirus or togavirus transmitted by mosquito bites
    - Endemic only in Africa and South America
    - Sudden onset of severe headache, photophobia, myalgias, and palpitations
    - Early tachycardia with late bradycardia and hypotension, jaundice, hemorrhagic phenomena (gastrointestinal bleeding, mucosal lesions) in the severe form
    - Proteinuria, leukopenia, hyperbilirubinemia
    - Virus isolated from blood; serologic tests positive after second week of illness

- ## Differential Diagnosis
    - Leptospirosis
    - Viral hepatitis
    - Typhoid fever
    - Biliary tract disease
    - Malaria
    - Dengue

- ## Treatment
    - Active immunization of persons living in or traveling to endemic areas
    - Supportive care

Influenza

- ■ **Essentials of Diagnosis**
    - Caused by an orthomyxovirus transmitted via the respiratory route
    - Abrupt onset of fever, chills, malaise, dry cough, coryza and myalgias; constitutional signs may be out of proportion to catarrhal symptoms
    - Epidemic outbreaks usually occur in the fall or winter; incubation period is 4 days
    - Virus isolated from throat washings; serologic tests positive after second week of illness
    - Often complicated by acute sinusitis, otitis media, and pneumonia

- ■ **Differential Diagnosis**
    - Other viral syndromes
    - Bacterial pneumonia

- ■ **Treatment**
    - Yearly active immunization of persons at high risk (eg, chronic respiratory disease, cardiac disease, health care workers)
    - Supportive care for established disease
    - Chemoprophylaxis for epidemic influenza A effective with amantadine
    - Avoid salicylates, especially in children (associated with Reye's syndrome)

8

Infectious Mononucleosis (Epstein-Barr Virus Infection)

- **Essentials of Diagnosis**
  - An acute viral illness due to EBV, usually occurs between the ages of 10 and 35
  - Transmitted by saliva; incubation period is 5–15 days or longer
  - Fever, sore throat, malaise, lymphadenopathy
  - Frequently maculopapular rash, splenomegaly
  - Leukocytosis and lymphocytosis with atypical large lymphocytes by smear; positive heterophil agglutination test (Monospot) by fourth week of illness; false-positive RPR in 10%
  - Splenic rupture, hepatitis, myocarditis, neuritis, and encephalitis may complicate

- **Differential Diagnosis**
  - Other causes of pharyngitis
  - Hepatitis or other causes of hepatitis
  - Toxoplasmosis
  - Rubella
  - Acute leukemia or lymphoma
  - Kawasaki syndrome
  - Hypersensitivity reaction due to carbamazepine

- **Treatment**
  - Supportive care only; fever usually disappears in 10 days, lymphadenopathy and splenomegaly in 4 weeks
  - Ampicillin apt to cause rash
  - Avoid vigorous abdominal activity or exercise

8

RICKETTSIAL INFECTIONS

Epidemic Louse-Borne Typhus (*Rickettsia Prowazekii*)

- ■ Essentials of Diagnosis
  - Transmission of *R prowazekii* is favored by crowding living conditions, famine
  - Headache, chills, fever, often severe or intractable
  - Maculopapular rash appears on fourth to seventh days on trunk and axillae, then extremities; spares face, palms, and soles
  - Conjunctivitis, rales, splenomegaly, hypotension, renal insufficiency, and delirium in some patients
  - Serologic confirmation by second week of illness
  - Brill's disease: recrudescence of disease after apparent recovery

- ■ Differential Diagnosis
  - Other viral syndromes
  - Pneumonia
  - Other exanthems

- ■ Treatment
  - Prevention with louse control
  - Vaccine available in some part of the world (not USA)
  - Tetracycline and chloramphenicol equally effective

Rocky Mountain Spotted Fever (*Rickettsia rickettsii*)

- ■ Essentials of Diagnosis
  - Infection follows exposure to tick bite in endemic area
  - Influenzal prodrome followed by chills, fever, severe headache, myalgias, occasionally delirium and coma
  - Red macular rash with onset between second and sixth days of fever; first on extremities, then centrally, may become petechial
  - Leukocytosis, proteinuria, hematuria
  - Serologic tests positive by second week of illness

- ■ Differential Diagnosis
  - Measles
  - Typhoid fever
  - Meningococcemia
  - Endocarditis
  - Gonococcemia
  - Ehrlichiosis

- ■ Treatment
  - Tetracyclines or chloramphenicol
  - Vaccine in development

8

Scrub Typhus (Tsutsugamushi Disease)

■ **Essentials of Diagnosis**

- Exposure to mites in endemic area of Southeast Asia, western Pacific, Australia
- Black eschar at site of bite with regional or generalized lymphadenopathy, malaise, chills, headache, backache
- Conjunctivitis and fleeting macular rash
- Pneumonitis, encephalitis, and cardiac failure may complicate
- Serologic confirmation by second week of illness

■ **Differential Diagnosis**

- Typhoid fever
- Dengue
- Malaria
- Leptospirosis
- Other rickettsial infections

■ **Treatment**

- Tetracyclines or chloramphenicol

8

Q Fever (*Coxiella burnettii*)

- ■ Essentials of Diagnosis
  - Infection following exposure to sheep, goats, or cattle
  - Acute or chronic febrile illness with severe headache, cough, and abdominal pain
  - Pulmonary infiltrates by chest x-ray; leukopenia
  - Serologic confirmation by third to fourth weeks of illness
  - Hepatitis, encephalopathy, extensive pneumonitis, or culture-negative endocarditis may occur

- ■ Differential Diagnosis
  - Pneumonia due to other causes
  - Viral or granulomatous hepatitis
  - Brucellosis
  - Other causes of endocarditis

- ■ Treatment
  - Tetracyclines suppressive but not always curative, especially with endocarditis
  - Vaccine being developed

BACTERIAL INFECTIONS

Streptococcal Pharyngitis

Strep. pyogenes (Gp. A)

- ■ Essentials of Diagnosis
  - Abrupt onset of sore throat, fever, malaise, nausea, headache
  - Pharynx erythematous and edematous with exudate; cervical adenopathy
  - Strawberry tongue
  - Throat culture or rapid antigen detection confirmatory
  - If erythrotoxin is produced, evanescent rash in groin and axillae, red and papular with petechiae and fine desquamation
  - Complications: glomerulonephritis, rheumatic fever

- ■ Differential Diagnosis
  - Adenovirus
  - Epstein-Barr virus
  - Diphtheria
  - Candidiasis
  - Necrotizing ulcerative gingivostomatitis
  - With rash: meningococcemia, toxic shock syndrome, drug reaction, viral exanthem

- ■ Treatment
  - For two or more clinical criteria (cervical adenopathy, fever, absence of runny nose, or exudate): empiric penicillin
  - If equivocal, await culture
  - If history of rheumatic fever, continuous antibiotic prophylaxis for 5 years recommended

Streptococcal Skin Infection

- **Essentials of Diagnosis**
    - Fever
    - Erysipelas: rapidly spreading cutaneous erythema and edema with sharp borders
    - Impetigo: rapidly spreading erythema with vesicular or denuded areas and salmon-colored crust
    - Culture of wound grows group A streptococci
    - Complications: glomerulonephritis

- **Differential Diagnosis**
    - Other infectious cellulitis (staphylococcal)
    - Toxic shock syndrome
    - Beriberi

- **Treatment**
    - Penicillin for culture-proved streptococcal infection
    - Staphylococcal coverage (dicloxacillin) for empiric therapy

8

Pneumococcal Infections

- **Essentials of Diagnosis**
  - Pneumonia characterized by initial chill, severe pleuritis, fever without diurnal variation; consolidation and lobar infiltrates
  - Leukocytosis, hyperbilirubinemia
  - Lancet-shaped, gram-positive diplococci on Gram-stained smear of sputum
  - Meningitis: rapid onset of fever, altered mental status and headache; cerebrospinal fluid polymorphonuclear leukocytosis with elevated protein and decreased glucose; Gram-stained smear of fluid positive in 90% of cases
  - Endocarditis, empyema, pericarditis, and arthritis may also complicate
  - Predisposition to bacteremia in children under 24 months of age or in asplenic or immunocompromised adults (AIDS or elderly)

- **Differential Diagnosis**
  - Pneumonia, meningitis of other cause
  - Pulmonary embolism
  - Myocardial infarction

- **Treatment**
  - Blood culture prior to antibiotics for toxic patients
  - High doses of penicillin (if meningitis or endocarditis suspected) or erythromycin (for penicillin allergy)
  - Prevention by pneumococcal vaccine recommended in adults over 50 with any serious medical illness, all patients with sickle cell disease, and all asplenic patients
  - Emergence of resistant strains may create difficulty in choice of antibiotics

8

Staphylococcal Soft Tissue or Skin Infections

- ■ Essentials of Diagnosis
  - • Painful, pruritic erythematous rash with golden crusts or discharge
  - • Folliculitis, furunculosis, carbuncle, abscess, and cellulitis all seen
  - • Culture of wound or abscess is diagnostic; Gram-stained smear positive for gram-positive cocci *(Staphylococcus aureus)* in clusters

- ■ Differential Diagnosis
  - • Streptococcal skin infections

- ■ Treatment
  - • Penicillinase-resistant penicillin or cephalosporin; erythromycin may also be effective
  - • Drainage of abscess
  - • Positive blood culture raises possibility of endocarditis, osteomyelitis, or occult abscess

8

Staphylococcus Aureus-Associated Toxic Shock Syndrome

- ■ Essentials of Diagnosis
  - Abrupt onset of fever, vomiting, diarrhea, sore throat, headache, myalgia
  - Toxic appearance; often tachycardiac or hypotensive
  - Diffuse maculopapular erythematous rash with desquamation on the palms and soles; nonpurulent conjunctivitis
  - Association with tampon use; culture of nasopharynx, vagina, rectum, and wounds may yield staphylococci; blood cultures usually negative
  - Usually caused by toxic shock syndrome toxin-1 (TSST-1)

- ■ Differential Diagnosis
  - Streptococcal infection
  - Sepsis from other causes
  - Meningococcemia
  - Dengue
  - Rickettsial diseases

- ■ Treatment
  - Aggressive supportive care
  - Antistaphylococcal antibiotics to eliminate source

8

Clostridial Myonecrosis (Gas Gangrene)

- ■ Essentials of Diagnosis
  - Sudden onset of pain, swelling in an area of wound contamination
  - Brown or blood-tinged watery exudate with surrounding skin discoloration
  - Gas in tissue by palpation or x-ray
  - *Clostridium perfringens* in anaerobic culture or smear of exudate

- ■ Differential Diagnosis
  - Other gas-forming infections (mixed aerobic and anaerobic enteric organisms)

- ■ Treatment
  - Surgical debridement and exposure of infected areas
  - Hyperbaric oxygen of uncertain benefit
  - Intravenous penicillin
  - Appropriate tetanus prophylaxis

8

Tetanus (*Clostridium tetani*)

- ■ Essentials of Diagnosis
  - • Jaw stiffness followed by spasms (trismus)
  - • Stiffness of neck or other muscles, dysphagia, irritability, hyper-reflexia; late, painful convulsions precipitated by minimal stimuli
  - • History of nondebrided wound or contamination may or may not be obtained

- ■ Differential Diagnosis
  - • Infectious meningitis
  - • Rabies
  - • Strychnine poisoning
  - • Phenothiazine toxicity

- ■ Treatment
  - • Active immunization preventive
  - • Passive immunization with tetanus immune globulin and concurrent active immunization for all suspected cases
  - • Chlorpromazine or diazepam for spasms or convulsions, with additional sedation by barbiturates necessary in some cases
  - • Aggressive supportive care with attention to airway and laryngospasm
  - • Penicillin

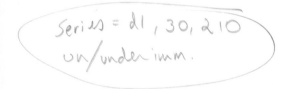

Series = d1, 30, 210
un/under imm.

Botulism (*Clostridium botulinum*)

■ Essentials of Diagnosis
- Sudden onset of cranial nerve paralysis, diplopia, dry mouth, dysphagia, dysphonia, and progressive muscle weakness
- In infants, irritability, weakness, and hypotonicity
- History of recent ingestion of home-canned, smoked, or vacuum-packed foods
- Demonstration of toxin in serum or food

■ Differential Diagnosis
- Bulbar poliomyelitis
- Myasthenia gravis
- Posterior cerebral circulation ischemia
- Tick paralysis
- Guillain-Barré syndrome

■ Treatment
- Removal of unabsorbed toxin from gut as soon as possible after ingestion
- Specific antitoxin; CDC may provide information about availability
- Aggressive support, including attention to respiratory function

Anthrax (*Bacillus anthracis*)

- ■ Essentials of Diagnosis
    - History of industrial or agricultural exposure (farmer, veterinarian, tannery or wool worker)
    - Persistent necrotic ulcer on exposed surface
    - Inhalation of spores causes severe tracheobronchitis and pneumonia with dyspnea and cough
    - Hematologic spread with cardiovascular collapse may complicate either cutaneous or pulmonary form
    - Confirmation of diagnosis by culture or specific fluorescent antibody test

- ■ Differential Diagnosis
    - Skin lesions: staphylococcal or streptococcal infection
    - Pulmonary disease: tuberculosis, fungal infection, sarcoidosis, lymphoma with mediastinal adenopathy

- ■ Treatment
    - Penicillin

8

Diphtheria (*Corynebacterium diphtheriae*)

■ Essentials of Diagnosis

- An acute infection spread by respiratory secretions
- Sore throat, rhinorrhea, hoarseness, malaise, fever (usually < 37.8°C)
- Tenacious gray membrane at portal of entry
- Smear and culture confirm Diagnosis
- Myocarditis and neuropathy may complicate, due to an exotoxin

■ Differential Diagnosis

- Other causes of pharyngitis (streptococcal, infectious mononucleosis, adenovirus)
- Necrotizing gingivostomatitis
- Candidiasis
- Myocarditis from other causes
- Poliomyelitis
- Myasthenia gravis
- Botulism

■ Treatment

- Active immunization (usually as DTP) is preventive
- Diphtheria antitoxin
- Penicillin or erythromycin
- Corticosteroids in selected patients with severe laryngeal involvement or myocarditis or neuritis
- Exposures of susceptible individuals call for booster toxoid, active immunization, antibiotics, and daily throat inspections

Pertussis (Whooping Cough)

- ■ Essentials of Diagnosis
    - An acute infection (*Bordetella pertussis*) of the respiratory tract spread by respiratory droplets
    - Two-week prodromal catarrhal stage of malaise, cough, coryza, and anorexia; predominantly in infants under age 2
    - Paroxysmal cough ending in high-pitched inspiratory "whoop"
    - Absolute lymphocytosis with extremely high white counts possible
    - Culture confirms diagnosis

- ■ Differential Diagnosis
    - Viral pneumonia
    - Foreign body aspiration
    - Acute bronchitis
    - Acute leukemia (when leukocytosis marked)

- ■ Treatment
    - Active immunization preventive
    - Erythromycin with hyperimmune gamma globulin in selected patients
    - Treat secondary pneumonia and other complications

8

Meningococcal Meningitis

- ■ Essentials of Diagnosis
  - Fever, headache, vomiting, confusion, delirium, or convulsions; often epidemic
  - Petechial rash of skin and mucous membranes
  - Positive Kernig and Brudzinski signs
  - Purulent spinal fluid with gram-negative intra- and extra-cellular organisms by Gram-stained smear
  - Culture of cerebrospinal fluid, blood, or petechial aspirate confirms Diagnosis
  - Disseminated intravascular coagulation and shock may complicate

- ■ Differential Diagnosis
  - Meningitis due to other causes
  - Petechial rash due to rickettsial, viral, or other bacterial infection
  - Thrombocytopenic purpura

- ■ Treatment
  - Active immunization for groups A and C available for selected susceptible groups (eg, military recruits)
  - Penicillin or chloramphenicol
  - Mannitol and corticosteroids for elevated endocranial pressure
  - Rifampin therapy for exposures

Legionnaire's Disease

- **Essentials of Diagnosis**
  - Classically caused by *Legionella pneumophila,* a common cause of community-acquired pneumonia in some areas
  - Usually in patients who are immunocompromised or have chronic lung disease
  - Malaise, dry cough, fever, headache, pleuritic chest pain, "toxic" appearance, purulent sputum
  - Chest x-ray with focal, patchy infiltrates often unimpressive early; later development of effusion or multiple lobar involvement common
  - Purulent sputum without organisms seen by Gram stain; diagnosis confirmed by culture or special silver stains or direct fluorescent antibodies

- **Differential Diagnosis**
  - Other infectious pneumonias
  - Pulmonary embolism
  - Pleurodynia
  - Myocardial infarction

- **Treatment**
  - Erythromycin, with rifampin added in severe disease or immunocompromised patients
  - Azithromycin and clarithromycin are also effective (but expensive) alternatives

Enteric Fever (Typhoid Fever)

- ■ Essentials of Diagnosis
  - A clinical syndrome due to any *Salmonella* species; the term "typhoid fever" is used when serotype *S typhi* is the cause and when accompanied by bacteremia
  - Transmitted by contaminated food or drink; incubation period is 5–14 days
  - Gradual onset of malaise, headache, sore throat, cough, followed by diarrhea or constipation; stepladder rise of fever to maximum of 40°C over 7–10 days, then slow return to normal
  - Rose spots, relative bradycardia, splenomegaly, abdominal distention and tenderness
  - Leukopenia; blood, stool, and urine culture positive for *S typhi* (group D) or other salmonellae

- ■ Differential Diagnosis
  - Tuberculosis
  - Infectious endocarditis
  - Brucellosis
  - Q fever and other rickettsial infections
  - Yersiniosis
  - Hepatitis
  - Malaria
  - Amebiasis
  - Lymphoma

- ■ Treatment
  - Active immunization helpful during epidemics and for travelers to endemic areas or household contacts of carriers
  - Ampicillin, chloramphenicol, or trimethoprim-sulfamethoxazole
  - Ciprofloxacin may be best agent for eradication of carrier state
  - Cholecystectomy may be necessary for relapsers
  - Complications occur in 30% of untreated patients and include intestinal hemorrhage or perforation, cholecystitis, nephritis, and meningitis

8

Salmonella Gastroenteritis
(Various *Salmonella* Species)

- **Essentials of Diagnosis**
  - Most common form of salmonellosis is acute enterocolitis
  - Nausea, headache, meningismus, fever, diarrhea (with or without blood), abdominal pain, and bloating occurring 8–48 hours after ingestion of contaminated food or liquid
  - Positive fecal leukocytes
  - Culture of organism from stool, blood, or other specimens

- **Differential Diagnosis**
  - Viral gastroenteritis
  - Other dysenteric illness (*Shigella, Campylobacter,* amebic)
  - Food poisoning
  - Ulcerative colitis

- **Treatment**
  - Attention to dehydration or electrolyte disturbance
  - Antibiotics (trimethoprim-sulfamethoxazole, ampicillin, or ciprofloxacin) for infants, severely ill, those with sickle cell disease, those for whom bacteremia is suspected, or immunologically impaired

8

Bacillary Dysentery (Shigellosis)

- Essentials of Diagnosis
  - Diarrhea (often bloody), abdominal cramps, fever, malaise, delirium
  - Positive fecal leukocytes; organism isolated in stool or blood culture

- Differential Diagnosis
  - Dysentery due to other bacteria (especially *Salmonella*)
  - Viral gastroenteritis
  - Amebiasis
  - Ulcerative colitis
  - Food poisoning

- Treatment
  - Attention to fluid and electrolyte abnormalities
  - Antibiotics determined based on sensitivities of local Shigella species; trimethoprim-sulfamethoxazole or ciprofloxacin are the usual drugs of choice

Campylobacter Enteritis (*Campylobacter jejuni*)

- ■ Essentials of Diagnosis
  - Outbreaks associated with consumption of raw milk
  - Fever, vomiting, abdominal pain, bloody diarrhea
  - Fecal leukocytes present; presumptive diagnosis by darkfield or phase contrast microscopy of stool wet mount
  - Definitive diagnosis by stool culture

- ■ Differential Diagnosis
  - Shigellosis
  - Salmonellosis
  - Viral gastroenteritis
  - Amebic dysentery
  - Food poisoning
  - Ulcerative colitis

- ■ Treatment
  - Erythromycin or ciprofloxacin will shorten the duration of illness
  - Disease is self-limited but can be severe

Cholera (*Vibrio cholerae*)

- **Essentials of Diagnosis**
  - Acute diarrheal illness that can lead to death because of profound hypovolemia
  - Occurs in epidemics under conditions of crowding and famine; acquired via ingestion of contaminated food or water
  - Sudden onset of frequent, large-volume diarrhea
  - Liquid ("rice water") stool is gray, turbid, with blood or pus
  - Rapid development of marked dehydration, acidosis, hypokalemia and hypotension
  - History of sojourn in endemic area or contact with infected person
  - Positive stool culture confirmatory; serologic testing useful in first to second weeks

- **Differential Diagnosis**
  - Other dysenteric illness (shigellosis, salmonellosis, enterotoxigenic *E coli*)
  - Viral gastroenteritis
  - VIP-producing pancreatic tumor

- **Treatment**
  - Vaccination preventive for travelers to endemic areas
  - Aggressive replacement of fluid and electrolytes
  - Tetracycline and many other antibiotics may shorten duration of *Vibrio* excretion

8

Brucellosis (*Brucella* Species)

- ■ Essentials of Diagnosis
    - History of animal exposure (veterinarian, slaughterhouse worker) or ingestion of unpasteurized milk or cheese
    - Cattle, hogs, and goats are the principal reservoirs
    - Insidious onset of fatigue, headache, arthralgia, anorexia, sweating; fever may become chronic and undulant
    - Cervical and axillary lymphadenopathy, hepatosplenomegaly
    - Lymphocytosis but normal total white cell count; positive blood, cerebrospinal fluid, or bone marrow culture; serologic tests positive in second week of illness
    - Osteomyelitis, epididymitis, or endocarditis may complicate

- ■ Differential Diagnosis
    - Lymphoma
    - Bacterial endocarditis
    - Influenza
    - Tuberculosis
    - Q fever
    - Typhoid fever
    - Tularemia
    - Malaria
    - Other causes of osteomyelitis

- ■ Treatment
    - Combination antibiotic regimen required for 21-day course

Tularemia (*Francisella tularensis*)

- ■ Essentials of Diagnosis
  - History of contact with rabbits, other rodents, and biting arthropods (eg, ticks) in endemic areas; incubation period is 2–10 days
  - Fever, headache, nausea begin suddenly
  - Papule progressing to ulcer at site of inoculation
  - Enlarged regional lymphadenopathy, splenomegaly
  - Diagnosis confirmed by culture of ulcerated lesion, lymph node aspirate, or blood; serologic confirmation positive after second week of illness
  - The disease may be primarily cutaneous, ocular, pneumonic, or typhoidal

- ■ Differential Diagnosis
  - Cat-scratch disease
  - Infectious mononucleosis
  - Plague
  - Typhoid fever
  - Lymphoma
  - Various rickettsial infections
  - Meningococcemia

- ■ Treatment
  - Combination antibiotics required; streptomycin and tetracycline are usually used

8

Plague (*Yersinia pestis*)

- ### Essentials of Diagnosis
  - History of exposure to rodents in endemic area (eg, western and southwestern USA); transmitted to humans by the bites of fleas or contact with infected rodents; human-to-human transmission with pneumonic plague
  - Sudden onset of high fever, severe malaise, myalgias; marked systemic toxicity
  - Regional lymphangitis and lymphadenitis with suppuration of nodes (bubonic form)
  - Bacteremia, pneumonitis, or meningitis may complicate
  - Positive smear and culture from aspirate or blood culture

- ### Differential Diagnosis
  - Tularemia
  - Lymphadenitis with bacterial disease of extremity
  - Lymphogranuloma venereum
  - Primary or secondary syphilis
  - Other bacterial pneumonia
  - Typhoid fever
  - Various rickettsial disease

- ### Treatment
  - Combination antibiotics required (eg, streptomycin plus tetracycline)
  - Tetracycline prophylaxis for persons exposed to patients with pneumonic plague
  - Strict isolation of pneumonic disease patients

Gonorrhea (*Neisseria gonorrhoeae*)

- **Essentials of Diagnosis**
  - A very common communicable disease spread via sexual activity; incubation period is 2–8 days
  - Purulent urethral discharge (men); vaginal discharge rare (women); may be asymptomatic in both sexes
  - Disseminated disease causes intermittent fever, skin lesions (few in number and peripherally located), arthritis, and tenosynovitis involving the knee, ankles, and wrists
  - Purpuric skin lesions, conjunctivitis, pharyngitis, proctitis, endocarditis, meningitis may occur
  - Gram-negative intracellular diplococci on smear or culture from any site, particularly urethra, cervix, rectum, and pharynx

- **Differential Diagnosis**
  - Cervicitis or vaginitis—or urethritis—due to other causes
  - Other causes of pelvic inflammatory disease
  - Reiter's disease
  - Meningococcemia

- **Treatment**
  - Penicillin or ceftriaxone intramuscularly for suspected cases; single high dose oral ciprofloxacin also effective
  - Oral antibiotics for concurrent chlamydial infection also recommended, as is empiric treatment of sexual partners
  - Intravenous antibiotics required for salpingitis, prostatitis, arthritis, or bacteremia
  - Surveillance and counseling for other sexually transmitted diseases essential (eg, syphilis, HIV)

Chancroid (*Haemophilus ducreyi*)

- ■ Essentials of Diagnosis
  - A sexually transmitted disease with an incubation period of 3–5 days
  - Painful, tender genital ulcer
  - Inguinal adenitis with erythema or fluctuance and multiple genital ulcers often develop
  - Balanitis, phimosis frequent complications
  - Women have no external signs of infection

- ■ Differential Diagnosis
  - Other genital ulcers
  - Syphilis

- ■ Treatment
  - Appropriate antibiotic (azithromycin, ceftriaxone, erythromycin, or ciprofloxacin)
  - Surveillance and counseling for other STDs (eg, syphilis, gonorrhea, HIV)

8

Granuloma Inguinale
(*Calymmatobacterium granulomatis*)

- **Essentials of Diagnosis**
    - A chronic relapsing granulomatous anogenital infection; incubation period is 1–12 weeks
    - Ulcerative lesions on the skin or mucous membranes of the genitalia or perianal area
    - Donovan bodies revealed by Wright or Giemsa stain of ulcer scrapings

- **Differential Diagnosis**
    - Other venereal ulcers
    - Syphilis
    - Herpes simplex

- **Treatment**
    - Appropriate antibiotic (erythromycin or tetracycline) for at least 21 days
    - Surveillance and counseling for other STDs (eg, syphilis, gonorrhea, HIV)

Cat-Scratch Disease (*Bartonella henselae*)

- ■ Essentials of Diagnosis
  - History of cat scratch or contact with cats; may be forgotten by patient
  - Primary lesion (papule, pustule, conjunctivitis) at site of inoculation in one-third of cases
  - One to 3 weeks after scratch, symptoms of generalized infection appear (fever, malaise, headache) accompanied by regional lymphadenopathy
  - Aspirate from enlarged lymph node yields sterile pus
  - Biopsy of node shows histopathologic features consistent with cat-scratch disease; positive skin test; serology for bacteria will be positive
  - Disseminated form seen in immunocompromised patients

- ■ Differential Diagnosis
  - Tularemia
  - Plague
  - Lymphadenitis due to other bacterial infections
  - Lymphoma
  - Tuberculosis
  - Lymphogranuloma venereum

- ■ Treatment
  - Nonspecific; exclusion of similar diseases most important
  - Isoniazid, rifampin, or erythromycin in immunocompromised patients

Actinomycosis

- ■ Essentials of Diagnosis
    - Due to an anaerobic gram-positive rod (*Actinomyces* species) that is part of the normal mouth flora; becomes pathogenic when introduced into traumatized tissue
    - Chronic suppurative lesion of the skin (cervicofacial in 60%) with sinus tract formation; thoracic or abdominal abscesses seen; pelvic disease associated with intrauterine devices
    - Sulfur granules found in pus from lesions with gram-positive hyphae on Gram-stained smear
    - Elevated sedimentation rate; anemia, leukocytosis
    - Isolation of *Actinomyces* species or sulfur granule from pus by anaerobic culture

- ■ Differential Diagnosis
    - Other causes of cervical adenitis
    - Tuberculosis
    - Nocardiosis
    - Crohn's disease

- ■ Treatment
    - Penicillin with continued treatment for weeks to months after remission
    - Surgical drainage may be necessary

Nocardiosis

- ### Essentials of Diagnosis
    - *Nocardia asteroides* and *Nocardia brasiliensis*—aerobic soil bacteria that cause pulmonary and systemic disease
    - Malaise, weight loss, fever, night sweats, cough
    - Pulmonary consolidation
    - Lobar infiltrates, effusion by chest x-ray
    - Delicate branching, gram-positive filaments by Gram stain, weakly positive acid-fast staining
    - Identification requires culture
    - Disseminated form may occur with abscess in any organ (brain abscesses and subcutaneous nodules are most frequent)
    - Alveolar proteinosis, corticosteroid use, immunodeficiency predispose to disease
    - *N brasiliensis* causes a lymphangitis after skin inoculation

- ### Differential Diagnosis
    - Actinomycosis
    - Tuberculosis or atypical mycobacterial infections
    - Other causes of pyogenic abscesses
    - Lymphoma

- ### Treatment
    - Parenteral and then oral trimethoprim-sulfamethoxazole for many months
    - Surgical drainage and resection may be needed

Tuberculosis

- **Essentials of Diagnosis**
  - Most infections sub-clinical, with positive skin test only
  - Symptoms progressive, and include cough, dyspnea, fever, night sweats, weight loss, and hemoptysis
  - Post-tussic apical rales on auscultation
  - Apical fibronodular pulmonary infiltrate on chest film, with or without cavitation, is most typical
  - Commonest extra-pulmonary manifestations include meningitis, genitourinary infection, miliary disease, arthritis, with localized symptoms and signs

- **Differential Diagnosis**
  - Pneumonia of other cause; bacterial and fungal (Histoplasmosis, Coccidiomycosis) most similar
  - Other mycobacterosis
  - HIV infection (may be associated)
  - Prolonged fever of other cause
  - Urinary tract infection, oligoarticular arthritis of other cause
  - Carcinoma of the lung
  - Lung abscess

- **Treatment**
  - Four drug regimens to include isoniazid and rifampin
  - Attention must be paid to sensitivity patterns due to increasing prevalence of isoniazid-resistant strains

Leprosy (*Mycobacterium leprae*)

- ■ Essentials of Diagnosis
  - A chronic infection due to the *M leprae*
  - Pale, anesthetic macular (tuberculoid) or nodular and erythematous (lepromatous) skin lesions
  - Superficial nerve thickening with associated sensory changes; progression slow and symmetric (lepromatous) or sudden and asymmetric (tuberculoid)
  - Skin test negative (lepromatous) or positive (tuberculoid)
  - History of residence in endemic area during childhood; mode of transmission probably is respiratory
  - Acid-fast bacilli in skin lesions or nasal scrapings; characteristic histologic nerve biopsy
  - Lepromatous type occurs in patients with defective cellular immunity

- ■ Differential Diagnosis
  - Lupus erythematosus
  - Sarcoidosis
  - Syphilis
  - Erythema nodosum
  - Erythema multiforme
  - Vitiligo
  - Neuropathy due to other causes
  - Amyloidosis
  - Cutaneous tuberculosis
  - Scleroderma
  - Syringomyelia

- ■ Treatment
  - Combination therapy for several months, including dapsone, rifampin, and clofazimine

Lymphogranuloma Venereum
(*Chlamydia trachomatis* types L1–L3)

- ■ Essentials of Diagnosis
  - A sexually transmitted disease with an incubation period of 5–21 days
  - Evanescent primary genital lesion
  - Inguinal lymphadenopathy and suppuration, with draining sinuses
  - Proctitis; rectal stricture; systemic joint, eye, or central nervous system involvement may occur
  - Serologic tests positive in second to third weeks of illness

- ■ Differential Diagnosis
  - Syphilis
  - Genital herpes
  - Chancroid
  - Lymph node involvement with tularemia
  - Tuberculosis
  - Plague
  - Pyogenic infection
  - Cancer of rectosigmoid
  - Rectal stricture due to other causes

- ■ Treatment
  - Tetracyclines; erythromycin in pregnancy
  - Dilation or surgical repair of rectal stricture

8

Psittacosis (*Chlamydia psittaci*)

- **Essentials of Diagnosis**
  - Contact with infected bird 7–15 days before onset of symptoms
  - Rapid onset of fever, chills, malaise, headache, dry cough, epistaxis
  - Meningismus, erythematous macular rash (Horder's spots), splenomegaly, dry crackles, temperature-pulse dissociation
  - Slightly delayed appearance of signs of pneumonitis; culture-negative endocarditis may occur
  - Serologic diagnosis by second week of illness; organism rarely isolated by culture of respiratory secretions

- **Differential Diagnosis**
  - Other atypical pneumonias (viral, mycoplasmal, rickettsial)
  - Typhoid fever
  - Lymphoma
  - Hypernephroma
  - Tuberculosis
  - Other causes of culture-negative endocarditis

- **Treatment**
  - Tetracycline

8

Primary Syphilis (*Treponema pallidum*)

- ### Essentials of Diagnosis
    - History of sexual contact, often of uncertain reliability
    - Painless ulcer (chancre) on genitalia, perianal region, oropharynx, or elsewhere 2–6 weeks following exposure
    - Nontender regional adenopathy
    - Fluid expressed from lesion positive by immunofluorescence or darkfield microscopy
    - Serology positive in 60%

- ### Differential Diagnosis
    - Chancroid
    - Lymphogranuloma venereum
    - Genital herpes
    - Lymphadenitis of other causes
    - Lymphoma
    - Drug eruption
    - Reiter's syndrome

- ### Treatment
    - Benzathine penicillin, 2.4 million units intramuscularly
    - In pregnancy or penicillin allergy, erythromycin may be used
    - Herxheimer reaction may occur following treatment

Secondary Syphilis

- ■ Essentials of Diagnosis
  - Usually appears a few weeks to 6 months after development of a chancre
  - Fever, generalized maculopapular skin rash (including palms, soles, and mucous membranes)
  - Weeping papules (condylomas) in moist skin areas
  - Generalized tender lymphadenopathy
  - Meningitis, hepatitis, osteitis, arthritis, or iritis may occur
  - Many treponemes in scrapings of mucous membranes or skin lesions by immunofluorescence or darkfield microscopy
  - Serology is uniformly positive

- ■ Differential Diagnosis
  - Viral exanthems
  - Pityriasis rosea
  - Drug rash, especially erythema multiforme
  - Multiple organ involvement may mimic meningitis, hepatitis, arthritis, uveitis, nephrotic syndrome

- ■ Treatment
  - Same as for primary syphilis
  - If central nervous system disease present, treat as neurosyphilis

Late or Tertiary Syphilis

- ■ Essentials of Diagnosis
  - May occur at any time after secondary syphilis; occurs in one-third of untreated patients
  - May be asymptomatic
  - Infiltrative tumors of skin, bone, liver; vascular disease with aortitis, aortic aneurysms, and aortic insufficiency
  - Neurosyphilis, early latent: meningovascular, with evidence of basilar meningitis or vascular accidents
  - Neurosyphilis, late latent: with wide-based gait, abdominal or leg pain, bladder symptoms, and slowly progressive dementia; tabes dorsalis; general paresis; Argyll-Robertson pupil (miotic, nonreactive)

- ■ Differential Diagnosis
  - Primary or secondary malignancy in any organ in which a gumma is involved
  - Aortic insufficiency due to other causes
  - Pernicious anemia
  - Other causes of acute abdomen
  - Other causes of aseptic meningitis
  - Other causes of neurogenic bladder

- ■ Treatment
  - Lumbar puncture for patients with syphilis longer than 1 year or with peripheral titers > 1:32 (unless asymptomatic); HIV-positive; or with any neurologic signs
  - For asymptomatic patients, treat as for primary syphilis
  - For neurosyphilis by symptom or central nervous system abnormality: 10–14 days of parenteral penicillin
  - Repeat lumbar puncture to follow central nervous system abnormalities to resolution
  - Treatment in HIV neurosyphilis controversial

Relapsing Fever (*Borrelia recurrentis*)

- ■ Essentials of Diagnosis
  - History of exposure to ticks in endemic area
  - Abrupt fever and chills, nausea, headache, arthralgia lasting 3–10 days with relapse at intervals of 1–2 weeks
  - Tachycardia, hepatosplenomegaly, rash
  - Spirochetes seen on blood smear during fever; serologic diagnosis positive at second week of illness

- ■ Differential Diagnosis
  - Malaria
  - Leptospirosis
  - Meningococcemia
  - Yellow fever
  - Typhus
  - Rat-bite fever

- ■ Treatment
  - Single dose of tetracycline, erythromycin, or penicillin
  - Herxheimer reaction may occur after treatment

Rat-Bite Fever (*Spirillum minus*)

■ Essentials of Diagnosis

- History of rodent bite; one to several weeks after bite, the site becomes swollen, indurated, and painful
- Fever, chills, nausea, vomiting, rash, headache, myalgia, and arthralgia; symptoms relapse at 24- to 48-hour intervals
- Regional lymphangitis or adenopathy, splenomegaly
- False-positive RPR
- Diagnosis confirmed by serologic testing or Giemsa-stained dark-field examination of blood or exudate

■ Differential Diagnosis

- Streptobacillary fever
- Tularemia
- Leptospirosis
- Borrelliosis
- Rickettsial infection
- Brucellosis
- Relapsing fever

■ Treatment

- Penicillin or tetracycline

Leptospirosis (*Leptospira* Species)

■ Essentials of Diagnosis

- An acute and often severe infection transmitted to humans by ingestion of food and drink contaminated by the urine of the reservoir animal (rats, dogs, cattle, swine)
- Biphasic course of 2–3 weeks: initial phase of high fever, headache, myalgias, and conjunctival injection, followed by apparent recovery and then return of fever associated with meningitis
- Jaundice, conjunctival hemorrhages, meningeal signs, abdominal tenderness
- Renal insufficiency, acalculous cholecystitis may occur
- Variable renal function abnormalities, elevated creatinine phosphokinase level
- Culture of organism from blood in cerebrospinal fluid or from urine, or direct darkfield microscopy of urine or cerebrospinal fluid diagnostic
- Serologic tests positive after first week; rapid ELISA for IgM now available

■ Differential Diagnosis

- Aseptic meningitis due to other causes
- Hepatitis
- Lymphoma
- Cholecystitis due to other causes
- Hepatorenal syndrome

■ Treatment

- Early treatment with penicillin or tetracycline may shorten course
- Herxheimer reaction may appear after therapy
- Doxycycline effective as prophylaxis for exposures

Lyme Disease (*Borrelia burgdorferi*)

erythema migrans

- Essentials of Diagnosis
  - History of exposure to *Ixodes* species of tick in endemic area; most USA cases occur in the Northeast, upper Midwest, and along the Pacific Coast
  - Stage I: Cutaneous and local (flu-like syndrome, erythema chronicum migrans with flat macular rash and erythema with central clearing); usually occurs about 1 week after tick bite
  - Stage II: Neurologic (Bell's palsy, meningoencephalitis, aseptic meningitis, peripheral neuropathy, transverse myelitis)
  - Stage III: Musculoskeletal (arthritis, migratory polyarthropathy, frank arthritis, synovitis)
  - Large amount of clinical overlap between stages seen
  - Mild carditis may occur
  - Serologic diagnosis is possible after 2–4 weeks of illness; rarely, organism can be cultured from blood, cerebrospinal fluid, or rash aspirate

- Differential Diagnosis
  - Stage I: other causes of viral exanthems
  - Stage II: other causes of peripheral neuropathy, transverse myelitis, encephalitis, aseptic meningitis, Bell's palsy
  - Stage III: collagen-vascular disease
  - Other causes of myocarditis, arrhythmias, and heart block

- Treatment
  - Antibiotic chosen depends on stage of disease
  - Effective prophylaxis for potential exposures controversial

OspA . Abs
↳ kill spirochetes
in tick

8

PROTOZOAL INFECTIONS

American Trypanosomiasis
(Chagas' Disease; *Trypanosoma cruzi*)

- ■ Essentials of Diagnosis
  - • Most infected patients are asymptomatic; transmitted by reduviid insects in endemic areas (Latin America and southwestern USA); some cases laboratory-acquired
  - • Unilateral bipalpebral or facial edema, conjunctivitis, local lymphadenopathy (Romaña's sign)
  - • Hard, edematous, erythematous, furuncle-like lesion with local lymphadenopathy (chagoma)
  - • Intermittent fever, lymphadenitis, hepatosplenomegaly, signs and symptoms of myocarditis or meningoencephalitis occur later
  - • Cardiac disease with arrhythmias, right-sided congestive heart failure and gastrointestinal disease (megacolon or megaesophagus) are seen
  - • Trypanosomes in blood; isolation by animal inoculation or serologic testing confirmatory
  - • Disease may occur after 30-year latent period

- ■ Differential Diagnosis
  - • Trichinosis
  - • Kala-azar
  - • Malaria
  - • Congestive heart failure due to other causes
  - • Meningoencephalitis due to other causes

- ■ Treatment
  - • Nifurtimox effective during acute phase but less so in chronic stage
  - • Benznidazole effective (not available in the USA)
  - • Ketoconazole of uncertain benefit

Amebiasis (*Entamoeba histolytica*)

- ### Essentials of Diagnosis
    - Infection of the large intestine; the parasite may be carried to the liver, lungs, brain, or other organs
    - Recurrent bouts of diarrhea and abdominal cramps, often alternating with constipation
    - In fulminant cases, frank bloody dysentery
    - Colonic ameboma or liver abscess may occur without obvious association with dysentery
    - Leukocytosis, eosinophilia variable; fecal leukocytes present
    - Organism demonstrable in stools or aspirate of abscess, with hematophagous amebas diagnostic
    - Cysts in stools in quiescent infection
    - Serologic tests diagnostic in invasive disease (dysenteric or abscess)
    - Ultrasound and CT scan useful to image hepatic abscesses

- ### Differential Diagnosis
    - Other causes of acute or chronic diarrhea
    - Ulcerative colitis
    - Pyogenic liver abscess
    - Hepatoma
    - Echinococcal hepatic cyst

- ### Treatment
    - Metronidazole plus diloxanide or iodoquinol for nondysenteric colitis
    - Diloxanide or iodoquinol for asymptomatic intestinal infection
    - Chloroquine after metronidazole, diloxanide, or iodoquinol for clearing trophozoites or residual amebas from liver

Primary Amebic Meningoencephalitis (*Naegleria* Species; *Acanthamoeba* Species)

- ■ Essentials of Diagnosis

    Naegleria:
    - Upper respiratory syndrome followed by rapidly progressing, usually fatal meningoencephalitis
    - Generally young, healthy persons with history of swimming in soil-contaminated fresh water 3–7 days prior to onset of symptoms
    - Amebas with large, central karyosome in fresh wet mount of uncentrifuged cerebrospinal fluid; can be cultured

    Acanthamoeba:
    - Skin lesions and ulceration with multiple organ dissemination, uveitis, chronic keratitis, or a more insidious onset of severe meningoencephalitis
    - History of preexisting debilitating disease; immunosuppressed state; trauma to skin, mucous membranes, or eye usually present

- ■ Differential Diagnosis
    - Other causes of meningitis or encephalitis
    - Other causes of keratitis

- ■ Treatment
    - Amphotericin B, miconazole, and rifampin with marginal success for *Naegleria* infections
    - Systemic ketoconazole, topical antifungals of uncertain benefit for *Acanthamoeba* infections

Babesiosis (Piroplasmosis; *Babesia* Species)

- ■ Essentials of Diagnosis
  - Exposure to *Ixodes* ticks in endemic area
  - *B microti:* irregular fever, chills, headache, diaphoresis, malaise without periodicity with hemolytic anemia and hepatosplenomegaly
  - *B divergens:* high fever, toxic appearance, severe hemolytic anemia, liver and renal failure, with splenectomized patients particularly at risk
  - Intraerythrocytic parasite by blood smear diagnostic; serologic test is available

- ■ Differential Diagnosis
  - Malaria
  - Typhoid fever

- ■ Treatment
  - None specific
  - *B microti* infection usually benign and self-limited
  - *B divergens* infection usually fatal
  - Quinine and clindamycin, exchange transfusion of uncertain benefit in splenectomized patients

Coccidiosis (*Isospora belli; Cryptosporidium*)

- ■ Essentials of Diagnosis
  - An intestinal infection caused by one of three genera: *Isospora, Cryptosporidium,* and *Sarcocystis*
  - Watery diarrhea, crampy abdominal pain, nausea, low-grade fever, malaise
  - Negative fecal leukocytes
  - Usually self-limited disease over weeks to months but may be catastrophic or life-threatening in AIDS patients
  - Diagnosis with identification of parasite in feces or duodenal aspirate or biopsy (*Cryptosporidium* requires acid-fast stain)

- ■ Differential Diagnosis
  - Cholera
  - Infectious enteritis (eg, *Giardia*)
  - Infectious colitis
  - Ulcerative colitis

- ■ Treatment
  - Isosporiasis: sulfadiazine or trimethoprim-sulfamethoxazole; in AIDS patients, indefinite therapy necessary
  - *Cryptosporidium:* no consistently effective therapy available

Giardiasis

- **Essentials of Diagnosis**
  - Infection of the upper small intestine that occurs worldwide
  - Most infections asymptomatic
  - Acute or chronic diarrhea with bulky, greasy, or malodorous stools
  - Upper abdominal discomfort, cramps, distention
  - Negative fecal leukocytes
  - Cysts and occasionally trophozoites in stools; trophozoites in duodenal aspirate or biopsy
  - Malabsorption syndrome may be seen in chronic disease

- **Differential Diagnosis**
  - Gastroenteritis or diarrhea due to other causes
  - Mucosal small bowel disease such as sprue
  - Other causes of malabsorption, such as pancreatic insufficiency

- **Treatment**
  - Metronidazole
  - Tinidazole, quinacrine, or furazolidone also effective
  - Recheck stools to assure therapy

8

Visceral Leishmaniasis
(Kala-Azar; *Leishmaniasis donovani* Complex)

■ Essentials of Diagnosis

- A zoonotic disease transmitted by bites of sandflies; incubation period is usually 4–6 months
- Local, nonulcerating nodule at site of sandfly bite (often inapparent)
- Irregular fever (often biquotidian) with progressive darkening of skin (especially on forehead and hands), malaise, wasting, diarrhea
- Progressive and marked splenomegaly and hepatomegaly, generalized lymphadenopathy, petechiae, and generalized wasting
- Progressive anemia, thrombocytopenia, and leukopenia with lymphocytosis and monocytosis
- Leishman-Donovan bodies demonstrable in splenic, bone marrow, or lymph node smears or buffy coat blood smear; serologic tests diagnostic after second week of illness

■ Differential Diagnosis

- Malaria
- Lymphoma
- Brucellosis
- Schistosomiasis
- Infectious mononucleosis
- Leukemia
- Anemia due to other causes
- Tuberculosis
- Leprosy
- African trypanosomiasis
- Subacute infective endocarditis

■ Treatment

- Sodium stibogluconate
- Pentamidine, amphotericin B for treatment failures
- High fatality rate if not treated

Malaria (*Plasmodium* Species)

- ■ Essentials of Diagnosis
  - History of exposure to mosquitoes in endemic area
  - Paroxysms of periodic chills, fever, headache, myalgias, and sweating with delirium; periodicity of fever determined by species
  - Jaundice, hepatosplenomegaly
  - Hemolytic anemia, leukopenia with monocytosis, thrombocytopenia, and liver function test abnormalities
  - Characteristic plasmodia seen in erythrocytes in thick or thin blood smear
  - Serologic test not available for diagnosis of acute disease
  - Hepatic failure, hypoglycemia, pulmonary edema, acute tubular necrosis (blackwater fever) may complicate

- ■ Differential Diagnosis
  - Influenza
  - Typhoid fever
  - Infectious hepatitis
  - Dengue
  - Kala-azar
  - Leptospirosis
  - Borrelliosis
  - Lymphoma

- ■ Treatment
  - Chemotherapy determined by species and drug sensitivities of endemic area
  - Chemoprophylaxis for travel to endemic area: oral chloroquine with addition of primaquine after leaving endemic area; mefloquine if resistant falciparum malaria present

Toxoplasmosis (*Toxoplasmic gondii*)

■ Essentials of Diagnosis

- Fever, malaise, headache, sore throat, myalgia, blurred vision
- Rash, hepatosplenomegaly, cervical lymphadenopathy, <u>retino-</u>choroiditis, central nervous system abnormalities
- In <u>immunocompromised</u> patients, <u>brain abscess with focal neuro-logic abnormalities most common</u>; pneumonitis, myocarditis also occur
- Serologic test positive though inconclusive if no negative tests were previously documented
- Isolation of tachyzoite from fluids (cerebrospinal fluid), secretion, or tissue biopsies

■ Differential Diagnosis

- Other causes of space-occupying brain lesions (cancer, abscess, lymphoma)
- Other causes of encephalitis (herpes simplex, CMV, viral encephalitis)
- CMV infection
- Epstein-Barr virus
- Other causes of myocarditis
- Other atypical pneumonias
- Other causes of lymphadenopathy (sarcoidosis, tuberculosis, lymphoma)

■ Treatment

- <u>Pyrimethamine-sulfadiazine,</u> clindamycin, spiramycin all effective
- Corticosteroids useful adjuvant in ocular disease
- Indefinite therapy required for AIDS patients

HELMINTHIC INFECTIONS

Schistosomiasis (Bilharziasis; *Schistosoma* Species)

- ■ Essentials of Diagnosis
  - Acute: Katayama fever—fever, diarrhea, dry cough, urticaria; cercarial dermatitis—transient erythematous pruritic skin rash in areas of contact with water
  - Chronic: hepatosplenic—abdominal pain, anorexia, weight loss, hepatosplenomegaly, occasionally with ascites, bleeding esophageal varices; genitourinary—terminal hematuria, urinary frequency, urethral and bladder pain
  - Cor pulmonale may develop; portal hypertension, colonic or bladder polyps, spinal cord or brain complications seen—all due to eggs in the circulation
  - Demonstration of schistosome ova in stools, urine, or rectal biopsy diagnostic

- ■ Differential Diagnosis
  - Other causes of diarrhea
  - Cirrhosis
  - Hepatoma
  - Gastrointestinal neoplasm
  - Cystitis due to other causes
  - Genitourinary tumor
  - Transverse myelitis
  - Pulmonary hypertension due to other causes

- ■ Treatment
  - Chemotherapy dependent upon species and site of disease

Tapeworm Infections
(See also Echinococcosis and Cysticercosis)

- **Essentials of Diagnosis**
  - Six tapeworms frequently infect humans: *Taenia saginata* (beef tapeworm), *Taenia solium* (pork tapeworm), *Diphyllobothrium latum* (fish tapeworm), *Hymenolepis nana* (dwarf tapeworm), *Hymenolepis diminuta* (rodent tapeworm), *Dipylidium caninum* (dog tapeworm)
  - Usually asymptomatic but may cause nausea, diarrhea, abdominal cramps, malaise, weight loss
  - Segments found in clothing or on bedding
  - Megaloblastic anemia (*D latum*)
  - Characteristic eggs or proglottid segments of tapeworms in stool

- **Differential Diagnosis**
  - Diarrhea due to other causes
  - Malabsorption states due to other causes
  - Megaloblastic anemia due to other causes

- **Treatment**
  - Niclosamide for all infections except *H nana*
  - Praziquantel for *H nana* infections

8

Cysticercosis (*Taenia solium*)

- ■ Essentials of Diagnosis
  - Infection by the larval (cysticercus) stage of the *T solium;* locations of cysts in order of frequency are central nervous system, subcutaneous tissue, striated muscle, globe of eye, and, rarely, other tissues
  - History of exposure in endemic area
  - Seizure, headache, vomiting, blurred vision, fever
  - Focal neurologic abnormalities, papilledema, pear-shaped subcutaneous or muscular nodules
  - Eosinophilia; lymphocytic and eosinophilic pleocytosis with elevated protein and decreased glucose in cerebrospinal fluid
  - Parasite seen upon histologic examination of skin or subcutaneous nodule
  - Plain radiograph of soft tissue reveals oval or linear calcifications in nodules
  - CT or MRI of the head reveals calcification of cysts and signs of elevated intracerebral pressure
  - Serologic testing is helpful to differentiate from echinococcosis

- ■ Differential Diagnosis
  - Echinococcosis
  - Lymphoma
  - Toxoplasmosis
  - Brain abscess

- ■ Treatment
  - Praziquantel or albendazole
  - Treatment with steroids and mannitol for cerebral edema may be beneficial
  - Surgery in selected cases (orbital, retinal, spinal cord, or cisternal disease)

Echinococcosis (Hydatid Disease)

■ Essentials of Diagnosis

- A zoonosis in which humans are an intermediate host of the larval stage of the parasite
- History of close association with dogs in endemic area
- Often asymptomatic; signs of local obstruction or rupture and leakage (pain, fever, or anaphylaxis)
- Avascular cystic tumor of liver, lung, bone, brain, or other organs
- Eosinophilia; serologic tests positive after 2–4 weeks

■ Differential Diagnosis

- Bacterial or amebic liver abscess
- Tuberculosis
- Other lung, bone, or brain tumors
- Obstructive jaundice due to other causes
- Cirrhosis from other causes
- Anaphylaxis or eosinophilia from other causes

■ Treatment

- Surgical removal of cysts if location permits
- Albendazole (or mebendazole) may be effective if surgery not possible
- Treat pet dogs prophylactically (with praziquantel) if in endemic areas

8

Ascariasis (*Ascaris lumbricoides*)

- **■ Essentials of Diagnosis**
  - Pulmonary phase: fever, cough, hemoptysis, wheezing, urticaria, and eosinophilia; fleeting pulmonary infiltrates may be seen (Löffler's pneumonia)
  - Intestinal phase: vague abdominal discomfort and colic, vomiting
  - Inflammatory reactions in any organs and tissues invaded by wandering adult worms
  - Pancreatitis, appendicitis, intestinal obstruction may all complicate infection
  - Characteristic *Ascaris* ova in stool with larvae in sputum

- **■ Differential Diagnosis**
  - Pneumonitis due to other parasitic infiltrations (especially hookworm and *Strongyloides*)
  - Bacterial or viral pneumonia
  - Allergic disorders such as Löffler's syndrome, asthma, urticaria, allergic bronchopulmonary aspergillosis
  - Eosinophilic pneumonia
  - Pancreatitis, peptic ulcer disease, appendicitis, and diverticulitis due to other causes

- **■ Treatment**
  - Pyrantel pamoate
  - Piperazine and mebendazole are effective alternates

Enterobiasis (Pinworm; *Enterobius vermicularis*)

- ■ Essentials of Diagnosis
  - Nocturnal perianal and vulvar pruritus; insomnia, restlessness, and irritability
  - Children infected commonly
  - Vague gastrointestinal symptoms
  - Eggs of pinworms on skin or perianal area by cellulose tape test

- ■ Differential Diagnosis
  - Perianal pruritus from other causes (mycotic infections, allergies, hemorrhoids, proctitis, fissures, strongyloidiasis)
  - Enuresis, insomnia, or restlessness in children due to other causes

- ■ Treatment
  - Pyrantel pamoate drug of choice
  - Mebendazole also effective; do not give during pregnancy
  - Treat all household members

Hookworm Disease

- ■ Essentials of Diagnosis
  - Widespread in the moist tropics and subtropics; occurs sporadically in southwestern USA
  - Weakness, fatigue, pallor, palpitations, dyspnea, diarrhea, abdominal discomfort, and weight loss
  - Transient episodes of coughing or wheezing, with sore throat or bloody sputum sometimes seen
  - Pruritic, erythematous, maculopapular or vesicular dermatitis; deformed nails
  - Hypochromic microcytic anemia, eosinophilia
  - Guaiac-positive stool
  - Characteristic hookworm egg in stool

- ■ Differential Diagnosis
  - Iron deficiency due to other causes
  - Recurrent pulmonary embolism
  - Maculopapular or vesicular dermatitis due to other causes

- ■ Treatment
  - Pyrantel pamoate or albendazole
  - Mebendazole if ascariasis is also present
  - Iron supplementation for anemia

Strongyloidiasis (*Strongyloides stercoralis*)

■ Essentials of Diagnosis
- Pruritic dermatitis at sites of larval penetration
- Diarrhea, epigastric pain, nausea, malaise, weight loss, cough, rales and wheezing with chronic infection
- Transient or fleeting pulmonary infiltrates
- Eosinophilia; characteristic larvae in stool, duodenal aspirate, or sputum
- Hyperinfection syndrome: severe diarrhea with malabsorption, bronchopneumonia, gram-negative sepsis, often after corticosteroids given for "asthma"

■ Differential Diagnosis
- Eosinophilia due to other causes
- Recurrent diarrhea due to other causes
- Duodenal ulcer
- Asthma
- Recurrent pulmonary emboli
- Cholecystitis or pancreatitis due to other causes
- Intestinal malabsorption due to other causes

■ Treatment
- Thiabendazole or ivermectin
- Mebendazole, pyrantel pamoate, cambendazole, levamisole less effective

Trichinosis (*Trichinella spiralis*)

- ■ Essentials of Diagnosis
  - Vomiting, diarrhea, abdominal pain within first week of ingestion of inadequately cooked pork, boar, or bear
  - Second week characterized by muscle pain and tenderness, fever, periorbital and facial edema, conjunctivitis; splinter hemorrhages; symptoms due to dissemination of larvae
  - Eosinophilia and variably elevated serum CK, LDH, and AST; erythrocyte sedimentation rate low
  - Positive skin and serologic tests
  - Diagnosis confirmed by finding larvae in muscle biopsy

- ■ Differential Diagnosis
  - Dermatomyositis
  - Polyarteritis nodosa
  - Endocarditis
  - Diarrhea due to other infections

- ■ Treatment
  - Thiabendazole or mebendazole for intestinal phase
  - Corticosteroids during larval invasion and for systemic sequelae; they should not be used during the intestinal phase

8

FUNGAL INFECTIONS

Candidiasis (*Candida albicans*)

- ■ Essentials of Diagnosis
    - Plaque-like or ulcerative lesions of oral mucosa (thrush)
    - Vulvovaginitis, skin fold infections, or paronychia
    - Esophageal, pulmonary, central nervous system, or disseminated disease in immunosuppressed patients
    - Endocarditis in patients with prosthetic valves
    - A compatible clinical picture, susceptible host, and finding *Candida* in tissue specimens should establish diagnosis; positive blood cultures in absence of localizing findings may be difficult to interpret

- ■ Differential Diagnosis
    - Severe atopic dermatitis
    - Herpetic or cytomegalovirus esophagitis
    - Other fungal or basilar meningitides

- ■ Treatment
    - Nystatin, clotrimazole, miconazole for local lesions
    - Ketoconazole or fluconazole for systemic infections
    - Amphotericin B for severe infection

Histoplasmosis (*Histoplasma capsulatum*)

- ■ Essentials of Diagnosis
  - History of bird or bat exposure or of living near a river valley
  - Often asymptomatic; variable cough, fever, malaise, chest pain in self-limited infections
  - Ulceration of naso- and oropharynx, hepatosplenomegaly, generalized lymphadenopathy in disseminated disease
  - Skin test of limited value
  - Urinary histoplasma antigen is diagnostic; small budding fungus cells found in reticuloendothelial cells; biopsy and culture of organism confirms Diagnosis

- ■ Differential Diagnosis
  - Tuberculosis
  - Blastomycosis
  - Coccidioidomycosis
  - Lymphoma

- ■ Treatment
  - Oral itraconazole for most infections
  - Amphotericin B in severe disease or in those who have failed itraconazole treatment

Coccidioidomycosis (*Coccidioides immitis*)

- ■ Essentials of Diagnosis
  - Pulmonary form: fever, pleuritis, productive cough, anorexia, weight loss, erythema nodosum and erythema multiforme with arthralgias, "desert rheumatism"
  - Incubation period 10–30 days
  - Disseminated lesions involve skin, bones, and meninges
  - Eosinophilia and leukocytosis
  - Sporangia in pus, sputum, or cerebrospinal fluid may be seen
  - Radiographic studies show nodular pulmonary infiltrates with thin-walled cavities and hilar adenopathy
  - Skin test of limited value, but serologic testing is helpful both diagnostically and prognostically

- ■ Differential Diagnosis
  - Tuberculosis
  - Histoplasmosis
  - Blastomycosis
  - Osteomyelitis from other causes
  - Aseptic meningitis from other causes

- ■ Treatment
  - Amphotericin B for disseminated disease
  - Fluconazole or ketoconazole in mild disease

Cryptococcosis (*Cryptococcus neoformans*)

- ## Essentials of Diagnosis
  - Opportunistic disease seen most commonly in AIDS patients
  - Findings may be subtle, with headache, fever, photophobia, and neurologic signs
  - Meningeal signs with positive Kernig and Brudzinski; patellar and Achilles reflexes diminished
  - Solitary, local skin lesions may be seen
  - Subacute respiratory infection with low-grade fever, pleuritic pain, and cough seen as well
  - Spinal fluid findings include increased pressure, variable pleocytosis, increased protein, and decreased glucose
  - Large encapsulated yeasts by India ink mount of spinal fluid or cryptococcal antigen serology positive on both serum and spinal fluid

- ## Differential Diagnosis
  - Other causes of meningitis
  - Lymphoma
  - Tuberculosis

- ## Treatment
  - Amphotericin B for severe disease
  - Fluconazole can be used in many patients with or without flucytosine

Sporotrichosis (*Sporothrix schenckii*)

- **Essentials of Diagnosis**
  - Ulcer following trauma to extremity
  - Occupationally associated with exposure to plants or soil
  - Nodules found along lymphatic drainage which may ulcerate with a black eschar
  - Culture is needed to establish Diagnosis
  - Serology helpful in disseminated disease (rare)

- **Differential Diagnosis**
  - Tularemia
  - Anthrax
  - Other mycotic infections
  - Cutaneous tuberculosis

- **Treatment**
  - Itraconazole for several months is the treatment of choice for localized disease
  - Amphotericin B used in severe systemic infection
  - Potassium iodide solution orally in some cases

Pneumocystosis (*Pneumocystis carinii*)

[handwritten: Interstitial dz]

- **Essentials of Diagnosis**
  - Seen primarily in immunocompromised patients (AIDS, post tissue transplantation, lymphoreticular malignancy)
  - Fever, dyspnea, dry cough, often insidious onset
  - Dry crackles upon auscultation
  - Diffuse alveolar disease by chest x-ray _[handwritten: — NOT Lobar!]_
  - Increased A–a gradient; decreased DLco; elevated serum lactate dehydrogenase; abnormal gallium scan _[handwritten: ↳ ↑LDH]_
  - Organism identified by silver stain of secretions or biopsy
  - Atypical disease may be seen if patient is undergoing routine prophylactic therapy

[handwritten: Dx: bronchial lavage]

- **Differential Diagnosis**
  - Atypical pneumonia due to other causes
  - Congestive heart failure
  - Tuberculosis
  - Disseminated fungal disease
  - Kaposi's sarcoma

- **Treatment**
  - Many drug regimens effective; corticosteroids are adjunctive therapy if moderate or severe hypoxemia present
  - Chemoprophylaxis recommended for immunocompromised patients at risk _[handwritten: ↳ see p. 211]_

8

9

Oncologic Diseases

Carcinoma of the Larynx

- **Essentials of Diagnosis**
  - Most common between ages 50 and 70; occurs in heavy smokers, with alcohol as an apparent cocarcinogen
  - Early hoarseness in true cord lesions; sore throat, otalgia fairly common; odynophagia, hemoptysis indicate more advanced disease
  - Cosynchronous lung cancer in some patients
  - Lesions found at indirect laryngoscopy

- **Differential Diagnosis**
  - Chronic laryngitis, including reflux laryngitis
  - Laryngeal tuberculosis
  - Myxedema
  - Vocal cord paralysis due to laryngeal nerve palsy caused by left hilar lesion

- **Treatment**
  - Surgery and radiation therapy depending on result of staging
  - Role of chemotherapy for palliation is being defined

Colorectal Carcinoma

- ■ Essentials of Diagnosis
  - Altered bowel habits, rectal bleeding, bloody stools in left-sided lesions
  - In right colonic tumors: guaiac-positive stools, iron deficiency anemia
  - Palpable abdominal or rectal mass in minority
  - Characteristic barium enema or colonoscopic appearance; tissue biopsy is diagnostic
  - Elevated carcinoembryonic antigen (CEA) useful as marker of extent of disease though not helpful in diagnosis

- ■ Differential Diagnosis
  - Hemorrhoids
  - Diverticular disease
  - Benign colonic polyps
  - Peptic ulcer disease
  - Amebiasis, especially ameboma
  - Functional bowel disease
  - Iron deficiency anemia due to other causes

- ■ Treatment
  - Surgical resection for cure or palliation
  - Combination chemotherapy palliative for distant metastatic disease
  - Radiation with chemotherapy useful for rectal disease

Hepatocellular Carcinoma

- Essentials of Diagnosis
    - Most common visceral malignancy worldwide
    - Alcoholic cirrhosis, hepatitis B or C seropositivity, and hemo-chromatosis are risk factors
    - Abdominal enlargement, pain, jaundice, pruritus, weight loss
    - Hepatomegaly, abdominal mass; rub or bruit heard over right upper quadrant in rare patients
    - Anemia or erythrocytosis; liver function test abnormalities
    - Positive CEA and alpha-fetoprotein (AFP) helpful as markers of disease
    - Angiography with characteristic abnormality; CT or MRI delineates extent of disease; tissue biopsy is diagnostic

- Differential Diagnosis
    - Benign liver tumors: hemangioma, adenoma, focal nodular hyperplasia
    - Bacterial hepatic abscess
    - Amebic liver cyst
    - Metastatic tumor

- Treatment
    - Surgery for unicentric tumor may be curative in a minority of cases if uninvolved liver is normal histologically
    - Palliative systemic or intrahepatic arterial chemotherapy, hepatic arterial chemoembolization, and radiation of uncertain benefit
    - Transplant in carefully selected cases

9

Malignant Tumors of the Bile Ducts

- ■ Essentials of Diagnosis
  - • Jaundice, pruritus, anorexia, right upper quadrant pain
  - • Hepatomegaly, ascites, right upper quadrant tenderness
  - • Dilated intrahepatic bile ducts by ultrasound or CT scan
  - • Retrograde endoscopic cholangiogram characteristic; tissue biopsy is diagnostic
  - • Hyperbilirubinemia (conjugated), markedly elevated alkaline phosphatase and cholesterol
  - • Predisposing factors include choledochal cysts, primary sclerosing cholangitis, inflammatory bowel disease, *Clonorchis sinensis* infection

- ■ Differential Diagnosis
  - • Choledocholithiasis
  - • Drug-induced cholestasis
  - • Cirrhosis
  - • Chronic hepatitis
  - • Metastatic hepatic malignancy
  - • Pancreatic carcinoma

- ■ Treatment
  - • Palliative surgical bypass of biliary flow
  - • Stent bypass of biliary flow in selected patients
  - • Pancreaticoduodenectomy for resectable distal duct tumors curative in minority

9

Carcinoma of the Head of the Pancreas or of the Periampullary Area

- **Essentials of Diagnosis**
  - Peak incidence in seventh decade; more common in African Americans
  - Upper abdominal pain with radiation to back, weight loss, diarrhea, thrombophlebitis; painless jaundice
  - Palpable gallbladder or abdominal mass in some
  - Elevated amylase with liver function abnormalities; anemia, hyperglycemia, or frank diabetes in minority
  - Dilated common hepatic ducts by ultrasound or endoscopic retrograde cholangiogram
  - CT or MRI may delineate extent of disease and guide biopsy

- **Differential Diagnosis**
  - Choledocholithiasis
  - Drug-induced cholestasis
  - Hepatitis
  - Cirrhosis

- **Treatment**
  - Surgical diversion for palliation in most cases
  - Radical pancreaticoduodenal resection for disease limited to head of pancreas or periampullary zone (Whipple procedure) curative in rare cases
  - Radiation in selected patients for palliation

Carcinoma of the Female Breast

- ■ Essentials of Diagnosis
  - Increased in nulliparous or late childbearing women or those with family history
  - Painless lump; skin or nipple changes over breast occur later; axillary mass, malaise, weight loss are even later findings
  - Many found by mammography despite nonpalpable lump and absence of symptoms
  - Metastatic disease to lung, bone, or central nervous system may dominate presentation
  - Biopsy for histologic examination and hormone receptor status; bone scan, CBC, serum calcium, and chest x-ray required for staging

- ■ Differential Diagnosis
  - Mammary dysplasia (fibrocystic disease)
  - Benign tumor (fibroadenoma, ductal papilloma)
  - Fat necrosis
  - Mastitis
  - Thrombophlebitis (Mondor's disease)

- ■ Treatment
  - Surgical resection for cure with extent (lumpectomy versus modified radical mastectomy) dependent upon clinical setting
  - Additional radiotherapy required for cure in selected patients
  - Adjuvant chemotherapy in selected patients at high risk for metastatic disease
  - Palliative chemotherapy and radiation for metastatic disease
  - Hormonal manipulation depending on receptor status recommended for most patients, with ultimate role being defined

9

Carcinoma of the Male Breast

- **Essentials of Diagnosis**
  - Painless lump or skin changes of breast
  - Nipple discharge, retraction or ulceration, palpable mass, gynecomastia
  - Staging as in women

- **Differential Diagnosis**
  - Gynecomastia due to other causes
  - Benign tumor

- **Treatment**
  - Modified radical mastectomy with staging as in women
  - For metastatic disease, endocrine manipulation (physical or chemical castration) with tamoxifen, aminoglutethimide, or corticosteroids often quite effective

9

Cervical Intraepithelial Neoplasia (Dysplasia or Carcinoma in Situ of the Cervix)

- Essentials of Diagnosis
  - Asymptomatic in most
  - Cervix appears grossly normal with dysplastic or malignant cells by cytologic smear preparation
  - Culdoscopic examination with coarse punctate or mosaic pattern of surface capillaries, atypical transformation zone, and thickened white epithelium
  - Iodine-nonstaining (Schiller-positive) squamous epithelium is typical
  - Associated in some with human papillomavirus infection

- Differential Diagnosis
  - Cervicitis

- Treatment
  - Varies depending upon degree and extent of cervical or intraepithelial neoplasia; thus, staging crucial
  - Observation in mild dysplasia
  - Cryosurgery or CO_2 laser vaporization for moderate dysplasia
  - Cone biopsy or hysterectomy for severe dysplasia or carcinoma in situ

9

Cancer of the Cervix

- **Essentials of Diagnosis**
  - Abnormal uterine bleeding, vaginal discharge, pelvic or abdominal pain
  - Cervical lesion may be visible on inspection as tumor or ulceration
  - Vaginal cytology is usually positive; must be confirmed by biopsy
  - CT or MRI of abdomen and pelvis, examination under anesthesia useful for staging disease

- **Differential Diagnosis**
  - Cervicitis
  - Chronic vaginitis or infection (tuberculosis, actinomycosis)
  - Sexually transmitted diseases (syphilis, lymphogranuloma venereum, chancroid, granuloma inguinale)
  - Aborted cervical pregnancy

- **Treatment**
  - Radiotherapy valuable in all stages, with both intracavitary and external methods curative in limited invasive disease
  - Radical hysterectomy or pelvic exenteration for extensive disease not cured by radiotherapy

9

Endometrial Carcinoma

- ■ Essentials of Diagnosis
  - • Higher incidence in obesity, diabetes, nulliparity, and polycystic ovaries
  - • Abnormal uterine bleeding, pelvic or abdominal pain
  - • Uterus frequently not enlarged on palpation
  - • Endometrial biopsy or curettage is required to confirm diagnosis after negative pregnancy test; vaginal cytologic examination is negative in high percentage of cases
  - • Examination under anesthesia, chest x-ray, CT and MRI useful in staging

- ■ Differential Diagnosis
  - • Pregnancy
  - • Atrophic vaginitis
  - • Exogenous estrogen usage
  - • Endometrial hyperplasia or polyps
  - • Other pelvic or abdominal neoplasms

- ■ Treatment
  - • Hysterectomy and salpingo-oophorectomy for well-differentiated or localized tumors
  - • Combined surgery and radiation for poorly differentiated tumors, cervical extension, deep myometrial penetration, and regional lymph node involvement
  - • Radiotherapy for unresectable malignancies
  - • Progesterone for recurrence and for patients who are not candidates for surgery or radiation

9

Carcinoma of the Vulva

- ■ Essentials of Diagnosis
    - Prolonged vulvar irritation, pruritis, local discomfort, slight bloody discharge
    - History of genital warts common; association with human papillomavirus established
    - Early lesions may suggest chronic vulvitis
    - Late lesions may present as a mass, exophytic growth, or firm ulcerated area in vulva
    - Biopsy is necessary to make diagnosis

- ■ Differential Diagnosis
    - Sexually transmitted diseases (syphilis, lymphogranuloma venereum, chancroid, granuloma inguinale)
    - Crohn's disease with cutaneous fistulization
    - Benign tumors (granular cell myoblastoma)
    - Reactive or eczematoid dermatitis
    - Vulvar dystrophy

9

- ■ Treatment
    - Local resection for cases of in situ squamous cell carcinoma
    - Wide surgical excision with lymph node dissection for invasive carcinoma

Ovarian Tumors

- ■ Essentials of Diagnosis
    - Abdominal distention, pain, vaginal bleeding, weight loss
    - Ascites, abdominal mass
    - Ultrasonography or CT scan of the abdomen or pelvis is helpful to identify and delineate disease
    - Laparoscopy or laparotomy is necessary to obtain tissue from mass or ascites for cytologic examination
    - CA 125 (a tumor marker) is useful to monitor for recurrence, less valuable as a screening test

- ■ Differential Diagnosis
    - Uterine leiomyoma
    - Endometriosis
    - Tubal pregnancy
    - Pelvic kidney
    - Retroperitoneal tumor or fibrosis
    - Colorectal carcinoma
    - Chronic pelvic inflammatory disease (especially tuberculosis)
    - Metastatic pelvic tumor

- ■ Treatment
    - Premenopausal women with small ovarian masses can be observed with a trial of ovulation suppression for two cycles and repeat examination
    - Simple excision with ovarian preservation for many benign cell types
    - Unilateral salpingo-oophorectomy for certain cell types in younger women
    - Hysterectomy with bilateral salpingo-oophorectomy in post-menopausal women, those with bilateral disease, or those with extensive disease
    - Postoperative radiation for locally extensive disease
    - Combination chemotherapy for disseminated disease with variable results

9

Gestational Trophoblastic Neoplasia (Hydatidiform Mole & Choriocarcinoma)

■ Essentials of Diagnosis

- Uterine bleeding in first trimester
- Uterus larger than expected for duration of pregnancy
- No fetus demonstrated by ultrasound with sometimes characteristic findings of mole; excessively elevated levels of serum β-hCG for gestational duration of pregnancy
- Vesicles may be passed from vagina
- Preeclampsia seen in first trimester
- Thyrotoxicosis (from ectopic mole source) may occur as a rare complication

■ Differential Diagnosis

- Multiple pregnancy
- Threatened abortion
- Ectopic pregnancy

■ Treatment

- Suction curettage for hydatidiform mole
- For nonmetastatic malignant disease, single-agent chemotherapy (eg, methotrexate or actinomycin) very effective, but the role of hysterectomy is uncertain
- For metastatic disease, single-agent or combination chemotherapy depending upon clinical setting
- Follow quantitative β-hCG until negative and then frequently for surveillance of tumor recurrence

Thyroid Cancer

- ■ Essentials of Diagnosis
  - History of irradiation to neck in some patients; family history positive in medullary carcinoma
  - Often hard, painless nodule; dysphagia or hoarseness occasionally
  - Cervical lymphadenopathy when local metastases present
  - Thyroid function tests normal; nodule is characteristically stippled with calcium on x-ray, cold by radioiodine scan, and solid by ultrasound; does not regress with thyroid hormone administration

- ■ Differential Diagnosis
  - Thyroiditis
  - Other neck masses and other causes of lymphadenopathy
  - Thyroglossal duct cyst
  - Benign thyroid nodules

- ■ Treatment
  - Fine-needle aspiration biopsy best differentiates benign from malignant nodules
  - Total thyroidectomy for carcinoma; radioactive iodine postoperatively for selected patients with metastases; combination chemotherapy in anaplastic tumors
  - Prognosis related to cell type; papillary carcinoma enjoys excellent outlook, anaplastic the worst
  - Identification of responsible gene in medullary carcinoma allows thyroidectomy in presymptomatic patients

9

Carcinoma of the Prostate

- **Essentials of Diagnosis**
  - Symptoms of prostatism; bone (especially back) pain if metastases present; asymptomatic in many, however
  - Stony, hard, irregular prostate palpable in many
  - Osteoblastic osseous metastases visible by plain radiograph
  - Prostate-specific antigen (PSA) is age-dependent and may be elevated in older patients with benign prostatic hyperplasia (BPH); however, it reliably predicts extent of neoplastic disease, and recurrence after prostatectomy

- **Differential Diagnosis**
  - Benign prostatic hyperplasia (may be associated)
  - Scarring secondary due to tuberculosis or calculi
  - Urethral stricture
  - Neurogenic bladder

- **Treatment**
  - Radiation therapy or radical prostatectomy with pelvic node dissection for localized disease; nerve-sparing surgery in many allows continued potency
  - Radiation therapy for local nodal metastases in selected patients after prostatectomy
  - Hormonal manipulation of androgen activity for symptomatic metastatic disease

9

Tumors of the Testis

- ■ Essentials of Diagnosis
  - Painless testicular nodule; usually age < 40
  - Testis does not transilluminate
  - Gynecomastia, premature virilization in occasional patients
  - Tumor markers (AFP, β-hCG) useful except in pure seminoma

- ■ Differential Diagnosis
  - Genitourinary tuberculosis
  - Syphilitic orchitis
  - Hydrocele
  - Spermatocele
  - Epididymitis

- ■ Treatment
  - Orchiectomy, with lumbar and inguinal lymph nodes examined for staging
  - Additional radical resection of iliolumbar nodes indicated unless tumor is a seminoma for which radiation therapy is treatment of choice following surgery
  - Postsurgical radiation therapy also useful for other malignant cell types
  - Combination chemotherapy curative in many patients with metastatic disease

Carcinoma of the Bladder
(Transitional Cell Carcinoma)

- ■ Essentials of Diagnosis
  - More common in men over 40 years of age; predisposing factors include smoking and alcohol, as well as chronic *Schistosoma haematobium* infection in some areas
  - Usually asymptomatic; suprapubic pain, urgency, and frequency when concurrent infection present
  - Hematuria and anemia common; malignant cells by urine cytology
  - Tumor visible by cystoscopy

- ■ Differential Diagnosis
  - Other urinary tract tumor
  - Acute cystitis
  - Renal tuberculosis
  - Urinary calculi
  - Acute nephritis

- ■ Treatment
  - Endoscopic transurethral resection for superficial or submucosal tumors; intravesicular chemotherapy (with BCG, for example) reduces the likelihood of recurrence
  - Radiation therapy followed by cystectomy with urinary diversion for more invasive tumors
  - Radiation therapy for residual local disease; combination chemotherapy for distant metastases

Adenocarcinoma of the Kidney
(Renal Cell Carcinoma; Hypernephroma)

- ■ Essentials of Diagnosis
  - Gross or microscopic hematuria, back pain, fever, weight loss
  - Flank or abdominal mass may be palpable
  - Anemia in 30%, erythrocytosis in 3%; hypercalcemia, hypoglycemia sometimes seen
  - Renal ultrasound visualizes solid mass or renal and inferior vena cava clot or tumor

- ■ Differential Diagnosis
  - Polycystic kidney disease
  - Single complex benign renal cyst
  - Renal tuberculosis
  - Renal calculi
  - Renal infarction
  - Endocarditis
  - Prolonged fever of other cause

- ■ Treatment
  - Nephrectomy
  - Chemotherapy and radiation therapy for metastatic disease of marginal value; some authorities recommend resection of primary because of anecdotal reports of shrinkage of metastases

Malignant Tumors of the Esophagus

- **Essentials of Diagnosis**
  - Progressive dysphagia, initially during ingestion of solid foods, later with liquids; progressive weight loss and inanition ominous
  - Smoking, alcohol, asbestos are risk factors
  - Classic radiographic appearance with irregular mucosal pattern and narrowing, with shelf-like upper border or concentrically narrowed esophageal lumen
  - CT delineates extent of disease
  - Esophagoscopy with biopsy and cytologic study diagnostic
  - Squamous histologic picture predominates, associated with tobacco use, or stasis-induced inflammation (eg, achalasia); adenocarcinoma often associated with Barrett's esophagus related to chronic reflux

- **Differential Diagnosis**
  - Benign tumors of the esophagus
  - Benign esophageal stricture or achalasia
  - Esophageal diverticulum
  - Esophageal webs
  - Achalasia (may be associated)

- **Treatment**
  - Adjuvant chemotherapy with radiation therapy or surgical resection results in cure for only 10–15%
  - Dilation or radiation therapy for palliation of incurable disease

9

Carcinoma of the Stomach

■ Essentials of Diagnosis
- Few early symptoms; late complaints include dyspepsia, anorexia, nausea, early satiety, weight loss
- Palpable abdominal mass (late)
- Iron deficiency anemia, fecal occult blood positive; achlorhydria present in minority of patients
- Mass or ulcer visualized radiographically; endoscopic biopsy and cytologic examination diagnostic
- Associated with atrophic gastritis, *Helicobacter pylori;* role of diet, previous partial gastrectomy controversial

■ Differential Diagnosis
- Benign gastric ulcer
- Gastritis
- Functional or irritable bowel syndrome
- Other gastric tumors, eg, leiomyosarcoma, lymphoma

■ Treatment
- Surgical resection for cure; palliative resection with gastroenterostomy in selected cases
- Adjuvant chemotherapy may improve long-term survival in high-risk patients post surgery and may achieve remission in a minority of patients with metastatic disease

Bronchogenic Carcinoma

- **Essentials of Diagnosis**
  - Chronic cough, dyspnea; chest pain, hoarseness, hemoptysis, weight loss; often asymptomatic
  - Physical examination variable depending on stage of disease; localized wheezing, clubbing, superior vena cava syndrome may be observed
  - Enlarging mass, infiltrate, atelectasis, pleural effusion, or cavitation by chest x-ray; peripheral coin lesions in a minority
  - Diagnostic: presence of malignant cells by sputum or pleural fluid cytology or on histologic examination of tissue biopsy
  - Metastases to other organs or paraneoplastic effects may produce initial symptoms
  - Cigarette smoking most important cause, and concomitant asbestos exposure synergistic; also associated with second-hand smoke

- **Differential Diagnosis**
  - Tuberculosis
  - Pulmonary mycoses
  - Pyogenic lung abscess
  - Metastasis from extrapulmonary primary tumor
  - Benign lung tumor
  - Noninfectious granulomatous disease

- **Treatment**
  - Surgical resection for resectable non-small-cell carcinoma and all coin lesions irrespective of cell type; palliative chemotherapy and radiation for metastatic or nonresectable non-small-cell carcinoma
  - Combination chemotherapy and radiation for small-cell carcinoma

Pleural Mesothelioma

- ■ Essentials of Diagnosis
    - Insidious dyspnea, nonpleuritic chest pain, weight loss
    - Dullness to percussion, diminished breath sounds, pleural friction rub, clubbing
    - Nodular or irregular unilateral pleural thickening, often with effusion by chest radiograph; CT scan often helpful
    - Pleural biopsy usually necessary for diagnosis, though malignant nature of tumor only confirmed by natural history; pleural fluid exudative or hemorrhagic
    - Strong association with asbestos exposure, with usual latency from time of exposure 20 years or more

- ■ Differential Diagnosis
    - Primary pulmonary parenchymal malignancy
    - Empyema
    - Benign pleural inflammatory conditions (posttraumatic, asbestosis)

- ■ Treatment
    - No consistently effective therapy currently available, though investigations with combination surgery, radiotherapy, and chemotherapy are under way
    - One-year mortality rate > 75%

Primary Intracranial Tumors

- **Essentials of Diagnosis**
    - Many different tumors are included in this category (see below); the age predilections and prognosis vary depending upon the specific type
    - Half of all tumors are gliomas
    - Most present with generalized or focal disturbances of cerebral function; focal deficits depend upon the location of the tumor; generalized symptoms include nocturnal headache, seizures, and projectile vomiting
    - CT or MRI with gadolinium enhancement will define the lesion; posterior fossa tumors are better visualized by MRI
    - Biopsy is the definitive diagnostic procedure and will distinguish primary brain lesions from brain abscess and other intracranial space-occupying lesions such as metastases

    Specific types:
    - Glioblastoma multiforme: in strictest sense an astrocytoma, but rapidly progressive with a poor prognosis
    - Astrocytoma: More chronic course than glioblastoma, with a variable prognosis
    - Medulloblastoma: seen primarily in children and arises from roof of fourth ventricle
    - Cerebellar hemangioblastoma: patients usually present with disequilibrium and ataxia, with occasional erythrocytosis
    - Meningioma: compresses rather than invades adjacent neural structures; usually benign
    - Primary cerebral lymphoma: primarily seen with AIDS and other immunodeficient states

- **Differential Diagnosis**
    - Metastatic tumor
    - Brain abscess

- **Treatment**
    - Treatment depends upon the type and site of the tumor and the condition of the patient
    - Complete surgical removal may be possible if the tumor is extra-axial or is not in a critical or inaccessible region of the brain
    - Herniation treated with intravenous corticosteroids and mannitol
    - Prophylactic anticonvulsants are also commonly given

10

Fluid, Acid-Base, & Electrolyte Disorders

Dehydration (Simple & Uncomplicated)

- **Essentials of Diagnosis**
  - Dry mouth, thirst, oliguria
  - Decreased skin turgor, pinched facies, dry mucous membrane, tachycardia, postural hypotension
  - Impaired renal function, elevated urinary osmolality and specific gravity, decreased urinary sodium (fractional excretion of sodium is usually < 1%)

- **Differential Diagnosis**
  - Hemorrhage
  - Sepsis, burns, trauma, or surgery
  - Gastrointestinal fluid losses
  - Renal sodium loss
  - Adrenal insufficiency
  - Skin sodium losses associated with burns or sweating

- **Treatment**
  - Identify source of sodium loss if present
  - Volume replenishment with colloid, saline solution, or blood as indicated

Shock

- ■ Essentials of Diagnosis
  - History of hemorrhage, myocardial infarction, sepsis, trauma, anaphylaxis, or other overwhelming illness
  - Tachycardia, hypotension, hypothermia, tachypnea
  - Cool, sweaty skin with pallor; may be warm or flushed with early sepsis; clouded sensorium, altered level of consciousness, seizures
  - Oliguria, increased urinary osmolality and specific gravity, anemia, disseminated intravascular coagulation, metabolic acidosis
  - Hemodynamic measurements depend upon underlying cause

- ■ Differential Diagnosis
  - Numerous causes of the syndrome

- ■ Treatment
  - Correct cause of shock, ie, control hemorrhage, treat infection, correct metabolic disease
  - Restore hemodynamics, eg, hypovolemia, blood pressure
  - Maintain urine output
  - Treat contributing disease, ie, diabetes

10

Hypernatremia

- ■ Essentials of Diagnosis
  - Usually thirst; altered mentation, oliguria
  - Loose skin with poor turgor, tachycardia, hypotension
  - Serum sodium > 145 meq/L, serum osmolality > 300 meq/L
  - Excessive water loss (insensible) plus inability of patient to obtain water, ie, the very old, very young, critically ill, or neurologically impaired

- ■ Differential Diagnosis
  - Salt intoxication
  - Diabetes insipidus, either central or nephrogenic; drugs like lithium common cause of latter

- ■ Treatment
  - Rapid volume replacement followed by free water replacement over 48–72 hours
  - Desmopressin acetate for central diabetes insipidus

10

Hyponatremia

- **Essentials of Diagnosis**
  - Nausea, headache, weakness, irritability, mental confusion, generalized seizures
  - Lethargy, coma, and death may result
  - Serum sodium < 130 meq/L; osmolality < 270 meq/L; decreased uric acid if SIADH or primary polydipsia is the cause
  - May be in setting of hypovolemia (thiazide diuretics, renal disease, Addison's syndrome, fluid sequestration or third spacing), hypervolemia (congestive heart failure, cirrhosis, nephrotic syndrome), or euvolemia (hypothyroidism, SIADH, reset osmostat, primary polydipsia)

- **Differential Diagnosis**
  - Pseudohyponatremia (hyperglycemia, hypertriglyceridemia, paraproteinemia)

- **Treatment**
  - Treat underlying disorder
  - Corticosteroids empirically if Addison's syndrome suspected
  - Gradual correction (24–48 hours) of sodium unless central nervous system signs present
  - If hypovolemic, use saline
  - If hypervolemic, use water restriction, diuretics, and normal saline volume replacement of urine output

10

Hyperkalemia

- **Essentials of Diagnosis**
  - Weakness or flaccid paralysis, abdominal distention, diarrhea
  - Serum potassium > 5 meq/L
  - Electrocardiographic changes: peaked T waves, loss of P wave, sinoventricular rhythm, QRS widening, ventricular asystole, cardiac arrest

- **Differential Diagnosis**
  - Renal failure
  - Excessive potassium load
  - Acidemia
  - Primary hypoaldosteronemia (hyporeninism, potassium-sparing diuretics, ACE inhibitors, adrenal disease, interstitial renal disease)

- **Treatment**
  - Emergency: intravenous bicarbonate, calcium chloride, glucose and insulin
  - Dietary potassium restriction with sodium polystyrene sulfonate (eg, Kayexalate) or diuretic to lower body potassium subacutely
  - Dialysis if renal failure or severe acidosis complicates

10

Hypokalemia

- **Essentials of Diagnosis**
  - Muscle weakness, flaccid paralysis, lethargy, paresthesia, polyuria, anorexia
  - Hyporeflexia, weakness, ileus
  - Electrocardiographic changes: T wave flattening and ST depression → AV block → cardiac arrest
  - Serum potassium < 3.5 meq/L; metabolic alkalosis sometimes concurrent

- **Differential Diagnosis**
  - Severe dietary potassium restriction
  - Alkalosis, especially caused by gastrointestinal losses
  - Primary hyperaldosteronemia (adrenal disease, primary hyperreninism, and European licorice ingestion)
  - Diuretic use
  - Diarrhea
  - Magnesium depletion
  - Bartter's syndrome
  - Renal tubular acidosis (types I, II)
  - Hypokalemic periodic paralysis

- **Treatment**
  - Identify and treat underlying cause
  - Oral or intravenous potassium supplement

10

Hypercalcemia

- ■ Essentials of Diagnosis
    - Weakness, polyuria, dehydration, thirst
    - Anorexia, vomiting, constipation
    - Hyporeflexia, tremor, altered mentation, hypertension
    - Serum calcium > 10.5 mg/dL (correct with concurrent serum albumin)
    - Renal insufficiency or azotemia, decreased urinary specific gravity and osmolality
    - Shortened QT interval

- ■ Differential Diagnosis
    - Primary hyperparathyroidism
    - Malignancy (with secretion of parathyroid hormone-related protein)
    - Vitamin D intoxication
    - Sarcoidosis
    - Tuberculosis
    - Adrenal insufficiency
    - Hyperthyroidism
    - Immobilization
    - Familial hypocalciuric hypercalcemia

- ■ Treatment
    - Identify and treat underlying disorder
    - Volume expansion, loop diuretics
    - Glucocorticoids, calcitonin, plicamycin, bisphosphonates, and dialysis all useful in certain instances

10

Hypocalcemia

- ■ Essentials of Diagnosis
  - Abdominal and muscle cramps, dyspnea, tetany and convulsions
  - Positive Chvostek and Trousseau signs; cataracts in some cases
  - Serum calcium < 8.5 mg/dL (correct with concurrent serum albumin); hypomagnesemia may complicate; phosphate usually elevated
  - Electrocardiographic changes: increased QT interval

- ■ Differential Diagnosis
  - Hypoparathyroidism
  - Osteomalacia
  - Hypomagnesemia
  - Chronic renal failure
  - Hyperphosphatemia
  - Neoplasms treated with cytotoxic agent raising phosphate level

- ■ Treatment
  - Identify and treat underlying disorder
  - For tetany, calcium gluconate intravenously
  - Magnesium replacement if low
  - Oral calcium supplements
  - Phosphate-binding antacids if phosphate elevated

Hypermagnesemia

- **Essentials of Diagnosis**
  - Weakness, confusion
  - Bradycardia, hyporeflexia, altered mentation
  - Serum magnesium > 3 mg/dL; renal insufficiency usual; increased uric acid, phosphate, and decreased calcium seen
  - Increased PR interval → heart block → cardiac arrest

- **Differential Diagnosis**
  - Renal insufficiency
  - Excessive magnesium intake

- **Treatment**
  - Intravenous calcium chloride for severe manifestations (eg, electrocardiographic changes, respiratory arrest)
  - Volume expansion
  - Dialysis

10

Hypomagnesemia

- **Essentials of Diagnosis**
  - Muscle restlessness or cramps, athetoid movements, twitching or tremor, convulsions or delirium
  - Muscle wasting, hyperreflexia, positive Babinski and Chvostek signs, nystagmus, vertigo, ataxia
  - Serum magnesium < 1.5 meq/L, but symptoms usually require much lower level; decreased calcium, potassium often seen
  - Electrocardiographic changes: tachycardia, premature atrial or ventricular beats, increased QT interval, ventricular tachycardia or fibrillation

- **Differential Diagnosis**
  - Inadequate dietary intake (ie, malnutrition)
  - Malabsorption or diarrhea
  - Hypervolemia
  - Hyperthyroidism
  - Alcoholism
  - Loop diuretics, cisplatin, aminoglycosides

- **Treatment**
  - Identify and treat underlying cause
  - Intravenous magnesium replacement followed by oral maintenance
  - Calcium and potassium supplements if needed

Respiratory Acidosis

- ■ Essentials of Diagnosis
  - • Somnolence, confusion, dyspnea
  - • Respiratory distress, altered mentation, pulmonary abnormalities with or without cyanosis and asterixis
  - • Arterial P_{CO_2} increased; decreased arterial pH
  - • Severe lung disease may be acute (pneumonia, asthma) or chronic (COPD)
  - • Central to all is alveolar hypoventilation

- ■ Differential Diagnosis
  - • Chronic obstructive lung disease or airway obstruction
  - • Central nervous system depressants
  - • Structural disorders of the thorax
  - • Myxedema
  - • Ventilation-perfusion mismatch

- ■ Treatment
  - • Address cause
  - • Artificial ventilation if necessary to oxygenate

10

Respiratory Alkalosis

- ### Essentials of Diagnosis
    - Lightheadedness, numbness or tingling of extremities, circumoral paresthesias
    - Tachypnea; positive Chvostek and Trousseau signs; carpopedal spasm and tetany
    - Arterial pH > 7.45, P_{CO_2} < 30 mm Hg

- ### Differential Diagnosis
    - Restrictive lung disease or hypoxia
    - Sepsis
    - Liver disease
    - Salicylates
    - Pregnancy
    - Central nervous system lesion
    - Anxiety

- ### Treatment
    - Correct hypoxia or underlying ventilatory stimulant
    - Increase ventilatory dead space, eg, breathe into paper bag as in anxiety-induced hyperventilation

10

Metabolic Acidosis

- ■ Essentials of Diagnosis
  - Fatigue, hyperventilation, mental confusion, stupor or coma
  - Tachycardia, hypotension, shock, acetone breath
  - Arterial pH < 7.35, P_{CO_2} < 30 mm Hg, serum bicarbonate decreased; ketonuria; anion gap may be normal or high

- ■ Differential Diagnosis
  - Ketoacidosis (diabetic, alcoholic, starvation)
  - Lactic acidosis
  - Poisons (methanol, ethylene glycol, propyl alcohol)
  - Uremia
  - Diarrhea
  - Renal tubular acidoses

- ■ Treatment
  - Identify and treat underlying disease
  - Correct volume, electrolyte status
  - Intravenous bicarbonate rarely indicated

10

Metabolic Alkalosis

- **Essentials of Diagnosis**
  - Weakness, malaise
  - Hyporeflexia
  - Arterial pH > 7.45, P_{CO_2} > 45 mm Hg and serum bicarbonate > 30 meq/L; serum potassium and chloride usually low; increased anion gap seen

- **Differential Diagnosis**
  - Exogenous bicarbonate or base load
  - Loss of acid (vomiting or nasogastric aspiration)
  - Diuretic overuse
  - Primary hyperaldosterone states (hyperreninism, European licorice ingestion, adrenal tumor or hyperplasia, hypomagnesemia)

- **Treatment**
  - Identify and correct underlying cause
  - Replenish volume and electrolytes (use 0.9% sodium chloride)

10

11

Genitourinary & Renal Disorders

GENITOURINARY DISORDERS

Tuberculosis of the Genitourinary Tract

- **Essentials of Diagnosis**
  - Fever, malaise, night sweats, weight loss
  - Symptoms or signs of urinary tract infection may be present
  - Nodular, indurated epididymis, testes, or prostate
  - Variable pyuria or hematuria without bacteriuria ("sterile pyuria")
  - Culture of morning urine positive for *Mycobacterium tuberculosis*
  - Excretory urogram may reveal "moth-eaten" calices and beading of ureters
  - Ulcers or granulomas of bladder wall on cystoscopy

- **Differential Diagnosis**
  - Other chronic urinary tract infections
  - Interstitial nephritis
  - Nonspecific urethritis
  - Urinary calculi
  - Epididymitis
  - Bladder cancer

- **Treatment**
  - Standard combination antituberculosis therapy
  - Surgical procedures for obstruction, severe hemorrhage, or extensive destruction of the kidney ("autonephrectomy")

Bacterial Prostatitis

- ■ Essentials of Diagnosis
  - Acute bacterial prostatitis: fever, dysuria, urinary urgency and frequency, perineal or suprapubic pain; extremely tender prostate; leukocytosis, pyuria, bacteriuria, and hematuria
  - Caused by *Neisseria gonorrhoeae, Chlamydia trachomatis,* gram-negative rods (eg, *E coli, Pseudomonas*) or gram-positive organisms (eg, *Enterococcus*)
  - Prostatic massage is contraindicated (may produce septicemia)
  - Chronic prostatitis: older men, who may be asymptomatic; in some, urinary urgency and frequency, dysuria, perineal or suprapubic pain; prostate boggy, not tender
  - Expressed prostatic secretions demonstrate increased numbers of leukocytes; culture on occasion positive for gram-negative rods (eg, *E coli, Pseudomonas*) or *Enterococcus*

- ■ Differential Diagnosis
  - Urethritis
  - Cystitis
  - Epididymitis
  - Prostatodynia
  - Nonbacterial prostatitis
  - Perirectal abscess

- ■ Treatment
  - Symptomatic treatment with hot sitz baths and NSAIDs
  - For acute bacterial prostatitis in men under 35 years of age, treat for *N gonorrhoeae* and *C trachomatis* infection
  - For acute bacterial prostatitis in men over 35 years or homosexual men, treat for Enterobacteriaceae with oral or intravenous antibiotics (eg, trimethoprim-sulfamethoxazole or ciprofloxacin) for 21 days
  - For chronic bacterial prostatitis, oral antibiotics (eg, trimethoprim-sulfamethoxazole or ciprofloxacin) for 6–12 weeks

11

Urinary Calculi

- **Essentials of Diagnosis**
    - Sudden, severe colic, localized to the flank, commonly associated with nausea, vomiting, and fever; marked urinary urgency and frequency if stone lodged at ureterovesical junction
    - May be asymptomatic, however
    - Hematuria, pyuria with concurrent infection; presence of crystals in urine may be diagnostically helpful
    - Plain films of the abdomen, intravenous pyelography or sonography may be used to visualize location of stone
    - Depending on the metabolic abnormality, stones are composed of calcium oxalate, struvite, uric acid, or cystine; over 50% of patients develop recurrent stones

- **Differential Diagnosis**
    - Acute pyelonephritis
    - Chronic prostatism
    - Tumor of genitourinary system
    - Renal tuberculosis
    - Renal infarction

- **Treatment**
    - Stones usually pass spontaneously with analgesia and hydration
    - Antibiotics if concurrent infection present
    - Patient should save stone for analysis
    - Dietary change, thiazides, allopurinol, hydration, or a combination of these may be used to prevent recurrence, depending on composition of the stone
    - Lithotripsy or surgical lithotomy may be necessary in refractory cases

11

Acute Epididymitis

- ■ Essentials of Diagnosis
  - Sudden pain and swelling of epididymis, with fever, dysuria, urinary urgency, and frequency
  - Marked epididymal, testicular, or spermatic cord swelling and tenderness with symptomatic relief upon elevation of scrotum
  - Leukocytosis, pyuria, bacteriuria
  - Usually caused by *Neisseria gonorrhoeae* or *Chlamydia trachomatis* in men under age 40 and by Enterobacteriaceae in men over age 40
  - Ultrasound may be needed to differentiate from testicular torsion

- ■ Differential Diagnosis
  - Testicular torsion
  - Testicular tumor
  - Orchitis
  - Prostatitis
  - Testicular trauma

- ■ Treatment
  - Empiric antibiotics after culture of urine obtained
  - In men under age 40, treat for *N gonorrhoeae* and *C trachomatis* infection for 10–21 days
  - In men over age 40, treat for Enterobacteriaceae for 21–28 days
  - Analgesics and bed rest with elevation and support of scrotum

11

Testicular Torsion

■ Essentials of Diagnosis
- Sudden onset of severe, unilateral scrotal or inguinal pain
- Usually occurs in males under 25 years of age; may present as an acute abdomen
- Exquisitely tender and swollen testicle and spermatic cord; pain worsened with elevation
- Leukocytosis and pyuria
- Technetium 99m sodium pertechnetate scan shows decreased uptake on the affected side (versus increased uptake with epididymitis)
- Sonography confirms diagnosis

■ Differential Diagnosis
- Epididymitis
- Orchitis
- Testicular trauma
- Testicular tumor

■ Treatment
- Immediate surgery

11

Benign Prostatic Hyperplasia

- ■ Essentials of Diagnosis
  - • Urinary hesitancy, intermittent stream, straining to initiate micturition, reduced force and caliber of the urinary stream, nocturia, frequency, urgency
  - • Palpably enlarged prostate
  - • Hematuria, pyuria when infection complicates; high postvoid residual volume as determined by ultrasonography or excretory urography
  - • May be complicated by acute urinary retention or azotemia following prolonged obstruction

- ■ Differential Diagnosis
  - • Urethral stricture
  - • Vesicular stone
  - • Neurogenic bladder
  - • Prostate cancer
  - • Bladder tumor

- ■ Treatment
  - • Treat associated infection if present
  - • Minimize evening fluid intake
  - • Alpha$_1$-blockers for symptom relief
  - • Transurethral resection for intractable symptoms

11

RENAL DISORDERS

Acute Renal Failure

■ Essentials of Diagnosis
- Anorexia with nausea, lethargy, headache, confusion
- Azotemia with increased potassium and phosphate, decreased serum bicarbonate, appearing over days to weeks
- Oliguria in many (not all) patients
- Hematuria, mild proteinuria, isosthenuria (specific gravity of urine becomes fixed around 1.010, regardless of fluid intake); pericardial friction rub, asterixis may be present
- Kidneys of normal size or enlarged on imaging studies; anemia, renal osteodystrophy absent
- History of exposure to nephrotoxic agents, sepsis, trauma, surgery, glomerulonephritis, shock, or hemorrhage
- A low fractional excretion of sodium implies prerenal azotemia but may be seen in acute renal failure due to glomerulonephritis

■ Differential Diagnosis
- Prerenal azotemia (eg, hypovolemia)
- Intrinsic renal failure (eg, acute tubular necrosis)
- Postrenal azotemia (eg, obstructive uropathy)
- Chronic renal failure
- Hepatorenal syndrome

■ Treatment
- Identify and treat underlying disease or process
- Immediate volume resuscitation if hypovolemia present
- Supportive care for uncomplicated cases: minimize fluid intake, follow potassium and bicarbonate levels
- Role of diuretics uncertain; may convert oliguric renal failure to a nonoliguric process
- Dialysis for fluid overload, symptoms of uremia, hyperkalemia, acidosis, or pericarditis

11

Chronic Renal Insufficiency

- ■ Essentials of Diagnosis
  - Malaise, headaches, anorexia, nausea, hiccup, pruritus, polyuria, and nocturia
  - Hypertension, hyperpnea, pallor; signs of congestive heart failure common
  - Progressive azotemia over weeks to years
  - Anemia, azotemia, and metabolic acidosis; elevated serum potassium and phosphate, decreased serum calcium; isosthenuria (urine specific gravity fixed around 1.010); benign urinary sediment
  - Bilateral shrunken kidneys on imaging studies
  - End result of numerous glomerular or interstitial renal diseases

- ■ Differential Diagnosis
  - Obstructive uropathy
  - Acute renal failure
  - Prerenal azotemia
  - Drug toxicity

- ■ Treatment
  - Treat underlying disease and associated hypertension if present
  - Low-protein diet, salt and water restriction for patients with hypertension and edema, multivitamin and folic acid supplements; potassium, phosphorus, and magnesium restriction in most cases
  - Aluminum hydroxide for associated hyperphosphatemia; calcium and vitamin D supplements to prevent osteodystrophy
  - Dialysis (peritoneal or hemodialysis) for end-stage renal disease
  - Renal transplantation in selected cases

11

Acute Glomerulonephritis

- ■ Essentials of Diagnosis
  - Malaise, headache, fever, dark urine
  - History of preceding streptococcal or other infection or evidence of systemic vasculitis may be present
  - Hypertension, edema, and retinal hemorrhages may be present
  - Azotemia, moderate proteinuria, low urinary sodium, and hematuria with red cell casts
  - Depending on the history, additional laboratory abnormalities may include low complement levels (CH50, C3, C4), elevated antistreptolysin O (ASO) titer, elevated antideoxyribonuclease B (anti-DNA B) titer, anti-GBM antibody levels, anti-neutrophil cytoplasmic antibodies, and cryoglobulins
  - Renal biopsy in selected patients when therapeutic implications present

- ■ Differential Diagnosis
  - IgA nephropathy
  - Goodpasture's syndrome
  - Other vasculitides (eg, polyarteritis nodosa, SLE)
  - Infective endocarditis
  - Wegener's granulomatosis
  - Henoch-Schönlein purpura

- ■ Treatment
  - Treat underlying disease and associated hypertension if present
  - Supportive therapy with fluid and sodium restriction
  - Monitor for occasional severe complications (malignant hypertension, congestive heart failure, or rapidly progressive renal failure)

11

Nephrotic Syndrome

- ■ Essentials of Diagnosis
  - Anorexia, dyspnea, generalized swelling
  - Proteinuria (> 3.5 g per 24 hours), hypoalbuminemia (< 3.0 g/dL), edema, hyperlipidemia
  - Hypoalbuminemia may cause ascites, hydrothorax, anasarca and pulmonary edema
  - Lipiduria with oval fat bodies, and fatty and waxy casts in urinary sediment
  - Depending on the history, complement levels (CH50, C3, C4), serum and urine electrophoresis, antinuclear antibody (ANA), serologic tests for syphilis and hepatitis may be helpful
  - Renal biopsy may establish diagnosis, allow specific therapy
  - Increased incidence of hypercoagulability with peripheral venous thrombosis and renal vein thrombosis
  - May be primary or associated with systemic infections (eg, secondary syphilis, malaria, endocarditis), diabetes, multiple myeloma, heavy metals, and autoimmune diseases

- ■ Differential Diagnosis
  - Congestive heart failure
  - Cirrhosis
  - Constrictive pericarditis
  - Hypothyroidism
  - Hypertensive nephropathy

- ■ Treatment
  - Treat underlying systemic disease if present
  - Supportive therapy with fluid and sodium restriction, lipid-lowering agents
  - Low protein diet (unless urinary protein loss exceeds 10 g/24 h, at which point patients may need additional dietary protein to match losses)
  - Consider ACE inhibitor, especially if diabetes is present
  - Corticosteroids for minimal change disease (lipoid nephrosis); in focal and segmental glomerular sclerosis, membranous nephropathy, or membranoproliferative glomerulonephropathy, their use is less well established

11

IgA Nephropathy (Berger's Disease)

- **Essentials of Diagnosis**
  - Focal proliferative glomerulonephritis of unknown cause
  - Most common form of acute glomerulonephritis in the USA and Asian countries
  - Episodes of macroscopic hematuria, often associated with a viral infection, with or without gastrointestinal symptoms, over many years
  - Serum IgA increased in 30–50%; red cell casts may be seen; renal biopsy reveals inflammation and deposition of IgA with or without C3 in the mesangium of all glomeruli
  - Usually indolent but progressive renal disease often seen over 2–3 decades

- **Differential Diagnosis**
  - Poststreptococcal acute glomerulonephritis
  - Infective endocarditis
  - Goodpasture's syndrome
  - Other vasculitides (eg, polyarteritis nodosa, SLE)
  - Wegener's granulomatosis
  - Henoch-Schönlein purpura

11

- **Treatment**
  - Supportive therapy

Anti-Glomerular Basement Membrane Nephritis (Goodpasture's Syndrome)

■ Essentials of Diagnosis

- Triad of pulmonary hemorrhage, iron deficiency anemia, and glomerulonephritis due to anti-Glomerular Basement Membrane (GBM)
- Usually in young, white men who are smokers
- On immunofluorescence, renal biopsy reveals linear deposition of IgG with or without C3 deposits along the glomerular basement membrane
- Serum anti-GBM antibody is pathognomonic

■ Differential Diagnosis

- Wegener's granulomatosis, other pulmonary-renal syndromes
- Sarcoidosis
- Other vasculitides (eg, polyarteritis nodosa, SLE)
- Endocarditis
- Poststreptococcal acute glomerulonephritis

■ Treatment

- Plasmapheresis to remove circulating anti-GBM antibody
- Prednisone and cyclophosphamide may be useful
- Hemodialysis as necessary
- Renal transplant delayed until disappearance of antibody

11

Acute & Chronic Tubulointerstitial Nephritis

- ■ Essentials of Diagnosis
  - Responsible for 15% of cases of acute renal failure
  - Sudden decrease in renal function, associated with fever, maculopapular rash and eosinophilia; flank pain may be present
  - Hematuria, proteinuria, white blood cell casts and occasionally eosinophils in urine
  - Most drug-related (beta-lactam antibiotics or NSAIDs), but may be idiopathic or associated with infection
  - Chronic tubulointerstitial nephritis characterized by polyuria and nocturia, salt wasting, mild proteinuria, small kidneys, decreased urinary concentrating ability, hyperchloremic metabolic acidosis
  - May result from prolonged obstruction, analgesic abuse, chronic hypercalcemia, uric acid nephropathy, or exposure to heavy metals

- ■ Differential Diagnosis
  - Acute or chronic glomerulonephritis
  - Prerenal azotemia
  - Autoimmune disorders

- ■ Treatment
  - Discontinue all possible offending drugs or treat associated infection in patients with acute tubulointerstitial nephritis
  - Corticosteroids if renal function does not improve shortly after discontinuation of drug
  - Temporary dialysis may be necessary in up to one-third of patients with drug-induced acute interstitial nephritis
  - Relieve obstruction or discontinue analgesics in patients with chronic tubulointerstitial nephritis

11

Uric Acid Nephropathy

- **Essentials of Diagnosis**
    - Acute renal failure due to acute hyperuricemia and uric acid sludge; chronic renal failure due to long-standing hyperuricemia and uric acid stones
    - Patients undergoing chemotherapy for large tumor burden are at increased risk
    - Variable azotemia and urinary sediment; elevated serum uric acid; uric acid crystals in sediment do not correlate with renal insufficiency

- **Differential Diagnosis**
    - Acute glomerulonephritis
    - Renal failure of other cause
    - Prerenal azotemia
    - Nephrolithiasis of other cause

- **Treatment**
    - Intravenous hydration and alkalinization of urine
    - Pretreatment with allopurinol and intravenous hydration for selected patients receiving chemotherapy

11

Obstructive Nephropathy

- ■ Essentials of Diagnosis
  - Usually asymptomatic but may present with increasing malaise, nausea, and anorexia or acute suprapubic and flank pain; may or may not be symptoms of prostatism
  - Progressive azotemia
  - Renal ultrasound localizes site of obstruction with proximal tract dilation and hydronephrosis
  - Spectrum of causes include anatomic abnormalities, stricture, tumor, prostatic hypertrophy, drug effect, and neuromuscular disorders; 95% are postvesicular

- ■ Differential Diagnosis
  - Prerenal azotemia
  - Interstitial nephritis
  - Chronic renal failure due to any cause

- ■ Treatment
  - Urinary catheter for post vesicular obstruction
  - Urologic consultation for nephrostomy tubes if significant bilateral hydronephrosis present with bilateral ureteral obstruction
  - Treatment of concurrent infection
  - Observe for postobstructive diuresis

11

Myeloma Kidney

- **Essentials of Diagnosis**
    - Definition: Light chain immunoglobulins (Bence Jones proteins) directly toxic to tubules, or cause tubular obstruction by precipitation
    - May be initial presentation of multiple myeloma
    - Myeloma may also be associated with glomerular amyloidosis, nephrocalcinosis, nephrolithiasis, plasma cell infiltration of the renal parenchyma, hyperviscosity syndrome compromising renal blood flow and proximal or distal renal tubular acidosis
    - Serum and urinary electrophoresis reveals monoclonal spike in over 90% of patients

- **Differential Diagnosis**
    - Interstitial nephritis of other cause
    - Prerenal azotemia
    - Obstructive nephropathy
    - Nephrotic syndrome of other cause
    - Drug-induced nephropathy

- **Treatment**
    - Therapy for myeloma
    - Treat hypertension and hypercalcemia if present
    - Avoid contrast agents
    - Avoid dehydration and maintain adequate intravascular volume

11

Polycystic Kidney Disease

- ■ Essentials of Diagnosis
  - Inherited disease with autosomal dominant inheritance and nearly complete penetrance
  - Abdominal or flank pain associated with hematuria, frequent urinary tract infections, and positive family history
  - Hypertension, large palpable kidneys, positive family history
  - Renal insufficiency in 50% of patients by age 70
  - Diagnosis confirmed by ultrasonography or CT scan
  - Increased incidence of cerebral aneurysms, aortic aneurysms, and abnormalities of the mitral valve; 40–50% have concomitant hepatic cysts

- ■ Differential Diagnosis
  - Renal cell carcinoma
  - Simple renal cysts
  - Acquired polycystic kidney disease

- ■ Treatment
  - Treat hypertension and nephrolithiasis
  - Observe for urinary tract infection
  - Low-protein diet
  - High fluid intake
  - Excellent outcome with transplant

11

Renal Tubular Acidosis (RTA)

- ■ Essentials of Diagnosis
  - • Unexplained metabolic acidosis with a normal anion gap
  - • Type I (distal): inability to acidify urine, hypokalemia, abnormal (positive) urinary anion gap; may be familial (autosomal dominant) or secondary to autoimmune disease, obstructive uropathy, drugs (eg, amphotericin B), hypercalciuria, or sickle cell anemia
  - • Type II (proximal): bicarbonaturia, glycosuria, aminoaciduria, phosphaturia, and uricosuria due to impaired absorption; may be secondary to myeloma, drugs, or renal transplant
  - • Type IV: low renin and aldosterone; hyperkalemia, abnormal (positive) urinary anion gap; typical of diabetes mellitus, but drugs (eg, ACE inhibitors, NSAIDs), chronic interstitial nephritis, or nephrosclerosis may also be causative

- ■ Differential Diagnosis
  - • Fanconi's syndrome
  - • Diarrhea
  - • Hypokalemia or hyperkalemia from other causes

- ■ Treatment
  - • Discontinue offending drug or treat underlying disease if present
  - • Bicarbonate and potassium replacement for type I and type II RTA
  - • Fludrocortisone for type IV RTA

Acute Cystitis & Pyelonephritis

- ■ Essentials of Diagnosis
  - Dysuria with urinary frequency and urgency, abdominal or flank pain
  - Flank or suprapubic tenderness, fever, and vomiting with pyelonephritis
  - Pyuria, bacteriuria, hematuria, positive urine culture
  - Usually caused by gram-negative bacteria (eg, *E coli, Proteus, Klebsiella,* Enterobacteriaceae) but may be due to gram-positive organisms (eg, *Enterococcus faecalis, Staphylococcus saprophyticus, Staphylococcus aureus*)

- ■ Differential Diagnosis
  - Urethritis
  - Nephrolithiasis
  - Prostatitis
  - Pelvic inflammatory disease or vaginosis
  - Lower lobe pneumonia
  - Surgical abdomen due to any cause, eg, appendicitis

- ■ Treatment
  - Empiric oral antibiotics (eg, trimethoprim-sulfamethoxazole, cephalexin, or ciprofloxacin) for 3 days for uncomplicated cystitis
  - Oral or intravenous antibiotics (eg, fluoroquinolone or cephalosporin) for 14 days for pyelonephritis
  - Intravenous antibiotics and fluids if dehydration or vomiting present
  - Pyridium for early symptomatic relief
  - Hospitalize patients with diabetes, single kidney, or immunosuppression
  - Pursue evaluation for anatomic abnormalities in men who develop cystitis or pyelonephritis

11

Asymptomatic Bacteriuria

- ■ Essentials of Diagnosis
  - • Bacteriuria with absence of symptoms or signs referable to the urinary tract
  - • May be associated with obstruction, anatomic abnormalities, pregnancy, indwelling catheter, urologic procedures, or diabetes, but many patients have none of these, especially those in older age range
  - • Usually caused by Enterobacteriaceae, *Pseudomonas,* or enterococci
  - • History of recurring urinary tract infections may be present

- ■ Differential Diagnosis
  - • Drug-induced nephropathy, especially analgesics
  - • Renal tuberculosis
  - • Chronic renal failure from any cause

- ■ Treatment
  - • Indications for treatment include pregnancy, persistent bacteriuria, urologic procedures, after removal of indwelling catheter, and debatably diabetes mellitus
  - • Urine culture to guide antimicrobial therapy
  - • Surgical relief of obstruction if present
  - • In selected cases, chronic antibiotic suppression

11

12

Neurologic Diseases

Migraine Headache

- **Essentials of Diagnosis**
  - Onset in adolescence or early adulthood
  - Classic pattern: lateralized throbbing pain, with prodrome including nausea, photophobia, scotomas
  - May be triggered by stress, foods (chocolate, red wine), birth control pills
  - Basilar artery variant: visual disturbances, cranial nerve abnormalities, dysequilibrium, followed by occipital headache
  - Ophthalmic variant: Painless loss of vision, scotomas, usually unilateral

- **Differential Diagnosis**
  - Tension headache
  - Cluster headache
  - Stroke
  - Mass lesion, eg, tumor or abscess

- **Treatment**
  - Avoidance of precipitating factors
  - Acute treatment: ergotamine with caffeine, analgesics (preferably at onset of prodrome), sumatriptan
  - Maintenance therapy includes aspirin, propranolol, amitriptyline, ergotamine, clonidine
  - Veropomil, valproic acid may also be useful prophylactically in selected patients

Idiopathic Epilepsy

- **Essentials of Diagnosis**
  - Abrupt onset of paroxysmal, transitory, recurrent alterations of central nervous system function usually accompanied by alteration in consciousness
  - Family history may be present
  - Altered mentation, focal or generalized, prolonged, continuous motor convulsions in grand mal; altered mentation or focal abnormalities may persist for up to 48 hours postictally
  - Petit mal seizures may only be manifested as episodic inattention in children or adults
  - Characteristic EEG during seizures; often abnormal during interictal periods

- **Differential Diagnosis**
  - Seizures due to metabolic (alcohol, electrolyte disturbance, cocaine), vascular, infectious, neoplastic, or immunologic disease
  - Syncope due to other causes
  - Narcolepsy
  - Psychiatric abnormalities (hysteria, panic attack)
  - Cerebrovascular accident (when patient first seen postictally)

- **Treatment**
  - Phenytoin and valproic acid for most types of epilepsy
  - Phenobarbital may be helpful in patients unresponsive to phenytoin
  - In petit mal epilepsy, ethosuximide, valproic acid, and clonazepam are useful
  - Status epilepticus is treated as a medical emergency with intravenous diazepam and phenytoin; general anesthesia with barbiturates or halothane may be necessary in refractory cases

12

Stroke

- ▪ Essentials of Diagnosis
  - • History of atherosclerotic heart disease, hypertension, diabetes, or valvular heart disease with or without atrial fibrillation
  - • Sudden onset of neurologic complaint, variably including focal weakness, sensory abnormalities, vision change, language defect, or altered mentation
  - • Neurologic signs dependent on vessels involved: hemiplegia, hemianopia, and aphasia in anterior circulatory involvement; cranial nerve abnormalities, quadriplegia in posterior circulatory disease; hyperreflexia, Babinski signs in both
  - • Deficits persist > 24 hours; if resolution in < 24 hours, transient ischemic attack or other process is present
  - • CT of the head maybe normal in the first 24–48 hours, depending on cause; large hemorrhage visible immediately; MRI a superior imaging modality in posterior fossa disease

- ▪ Differential Diagnosis
  - • Primary or metastatic brain tumor
  - • Subdural or epidural hematoma
  - • Brain abscess
  - • Endocarditis
  - • Multiple sclerosis
  - • Any metabolic abnormality (ie, hypoglycemia)
  - • Neurosyphilis

- ▪ Treatment
  - • General supportive measures
  - • Anticoagulation immediately for stroke due to cardiac source emboli, after hemorrhage excluded by CT or MRI
  - • Aspirin for thrombotic stroke
  - • Carotid endarterectomy may be considered later in selected patients
  - • Rehabilitative efforts with control of contributing factors
  - • Thrombolytics under investigation

12

Intracranial Aneurysm & Subarachnoid Hemorrhage

- **Essentials of Diagnosis**
  - Asymptomatic until expansion or rupture; latter often preceded by headaches that resolve (sentinel headache)
  - Rupture characterized by sudden onset of severe headache, altered mental status, photophobia, nuchal rigidity, and vomiting
  - Focal neurologic signs unusual except for third nerve palsy with posterior communicating aneurysm
  - Deep T wave inversions on ECG characteristic, leukocytosis common
  - CT scan or bloody cerebrospinal fluid confirmatory; cerebral angiography indicates size, location, and number of aneurysms
  - Multiple in 20% of cases; associated with polycystic renal disease, coarctation of aorta

- **Differential Diagnosis**
  - Primary or metastatic intracranial tumor
  - Hypertensive intraparenchymal hemorrhage
  - Ruptured arteriovenous malformation
  - Vascular headache, migraine headache
  - Giant cell arteritis
  - Meningitis

- **Treatment**
  - Antifibrinolytic agents (aminocaproic acid) in selected patients; calcium channel blockers may also reduce neurologic deficits
  - Definitive therapy with surgical clipping of aneurysm if anatomy suitable and if patient's functional status is otherwise acceptable

12

Arteriovenous Malformations

- **Essentials of Diagnosis**
  - Congenital vascular malformations that consist of arteriovenous communications without intervening capillaries
  - Patients typically young (< 30) and normotensive
  - May present as seizures (often focal) or transverse myelitis (spinal cord site)
  - Initial symptoms include hemorrhage (intracranial and subarachnoid), epilepsy, headache, and focal neurologic complaints
  - Up to 70% of arteriovenous malformations bleed during their natural history, most commonly before the patient is 40 years old
  - CT of the brain suggests diagnosis; angiography characteristically diagnostic, but some malformations may not be visualized; MRI often helpful

- **Differential Diagnosis**
  - Seizures due to other causes
  - Hypertensive intracerebral hemorrhage
  - Ruptured intracranial aneurysm
  - Intracranial tumor
  - Meningitis or brain abscess
  - Transverse myelopathy due to other causes

- **Treatment**
  - Surgical excision if malformation accessible and neurologic risk not great
  - Intracranial embolization for larger or surgically unapproachable malformations

12

Brain Abscess

- ■ Essentials of Diagnosis
    - History of sinusitis, otitis, chronic pulmonary infection, or congenital heart defect may be present
    - Headache, focal neurologic symptoms, seizure often present; lumbar puncture potentially dangerous
    - Examination may confirm focal findings
    - The most common infecting organisms are streptococci, staphylococci, and anaerobes; *Toxoplasma* found in AIDS patients
    - Ring-enhancing lesion on CT scan
    - Angiographic evidence of a mass lesion creating a vascular halo

- ■ Differential Diagnosis
    - Primary or metastatic tumor
    - Cerebral infarction due to arterial or sinus thrombosis, embolus
    - Subdural empyema
    - Encephalitis
    - Metabolic encephalopathies
    - Neurosyphilis

- ■ Treatment
    - Intravenous broad-spectrum antibiotics (with coverage to include anaerobic organisms) may be curative if abscess smaller than 2 cm in diameter
    - Surgical aspiration through burr hole if no response to antibiotic drugs, either clinically or by CT scan

12

Pseudotumor Cerebri
(Benign Intracranial Hypertension)

■ Essentials of Diagnosis

- Headache, diplopia, nausea
- Papilledema, sixth nerve palsy
- CT scan shows normal or small ventricular system
- Lumbar puncture reveals elevated pressure and normal cerebrospinal fluid formula
- Associations include endocrinopathy (hypoparathyroidism, Addison's disease), hypervitaminosis A, drugs (tetracyclines, oral contraceptives), chronic pulmonary disease; often idiopathic
- Untreated pseudotumor cerebri leads to secondary optic atrophy and permanent visual loss

■ Differential Diagnosis

- Primary or metastatic tumor
- Neurosyphilis
- Brain abscess or basilar meningitis
- Vascular headache, migraine headache

■ Treatment

- Treat underlying cause if present
- Acetazolamide or furosemide to reduce cerebrospinal fluid formation acutely
- Repeat lumbar puncture with removal of cerebrospinal fluid
- Oral corticosteroids may be helpful; obese patients should be urged to lose weight
- Surgical therapy with placement of ventriculoperitoneal shunt in refractory cases

12

Parkinsonism

- **Essentials of Diagnosis**
    - Insidious onset in older patient of rigidity, bradykinesia, and progressive postural instability and in many cases pill-rolling tremor (3–5/sec)
    - Mask-like facies, seborrhea of skin common, cogwheeling of extremities on passive motion
    - Absence of tremor may delay diagnosis
    - Reflexes normal
    - Mild intellectual deterioration often noted

- **Differential Diagnosis**
    - Tremor due to other causes
    - Phenothiazine, metoclopramide toxicity
    - Hypothyroidism
    - Wilson's disease
    - Shy-Drager syndrome
    - Depression
    - Huntington's disease

- **Treatment**
    - Carbidopa-levodopa is most effective medical regimen in patients with definite disability; dose should be lowered if dystonias occur
    - Anticholinergic drugs and amantadine may be temporarily effective
    - Bromocriptine may be useful in allowing reduction of carbidopa-levodopa dose
    - Inhibition of monoamine oxidase B with selegiline (deprenyl) offers theoretical advantage of preventing progression if given early in course, but not yet established for this indication

12

Huntington's Chorea

- **■ Essentials of Diagnosis**
  - Onset at age 30–50, with gradual progressive chorea and dementia; death usually occurs within 20 years after onset
  - The gene responsible is located on chromosome number 4
  - Family history usually present (autosomal dominant)
  - The earliest mental changes are often behavioral
  - CT scan shows cerebral atrophy

- **■ Differential Diagnosis**
  - Sydenham's chorea
  - Multiple lacunar infarcts of subthalamic nuclei
  - Other causes of dementia

- **■ Treatment**
  - Principally supportive
  - Antidopaminergics (haloperidol) or reserpine may reduce severity of movement abnormality
  - Genetic counseling for offspring

12

Gilles De La Tourette's Syndrome

- ■ Essentials of Diagnosis
    - Motor and phonic tics, onset in childhood or adolescence
    - Compulsive utterances, often of obscenities, is typical
    - Hyperactivity, nonspecific EEG abnormalities in 50%

- ■ Differential Diagnosis
    - Wilson's disease
    - Focal seizures

- ■ Treatment
    - Haloperidol the drug of choice
    - Clonazepam, clonidine, phenothiazine, pimozide if intolerant or resistant to haloperidol

Multiple Sclerosis

- **Essentials of Diagnosis**
  - Patient usually under 55 years of age at onset
  - Episodic symptoms that may include sensory abnormalities, blurred vision, sphincter disturbances, and weakness with or without spasticity
  - Neurologic progression to fixed abnormalities occurs variably
  - Single pathologic lesion cannot explain clinical findings
  - Multiple foci best demonstrated radiographically by MRI
  - Finding of oligoclonal bands on lumbar puncture is nonspecific

- **Differential Diagnosis**
  - Neurosyphilis
  - Optic neuritis due to other causes
  - Primary or metastatic central nervous system neoplasm
  - Cerebellar ataxia due to other causes
  - Pernicious anemia

- **Treatment**
  - Steroids may hasten recovery from relapse
  - Treatment with immunosuppressants and plasmapheresis may be effective, but role is controversial
  - Beta-interferon reduces the annual exacerbation rate; Cop 1 (a random polymer-simulating myelin basic protein) may also be beneficial

12

Syringomyelia

- **Essentials of Diagnosis**
  - Characterized by destruction or degeneration of the gray and white matter adjacent to the central canal of the cervical spinal cord
  - Loss of pain and temperature sense with preservation of other sensory function; unperceived burning or injury to hands characteristic presentation
  - Weakness, hyporeflexia or areflexia, atrophy of muscles at level of spinal cord involvement (usually upper limbs and hands); hyperreflexia and spasticity at lower levels
  - Thoracic kyphoscoliosis common; associated with Arnold-Chiari malformation
  - CT myelogram, MRI confirm diagnosis

- **Differential Diagnosis**
  - Spinal cord tumor
  - Multiple sclerosis
  - Amyotrophic lateral sclerosis
  - Neurosyphilis
  - Degenerative arthritis of the cervical spine

- **Treatment**
  - Laminectomy with needle aspiration of syrinx
  - Posterior myelotomy in selected cases

12

Guillain-Barré Syndrome
(Acute Idiopathic Polyneuropathy)

- ■ Essentials of Diagnosis
  - Progressive, often ascending, symmetric weakness with variable paresthesia or dysesthesia; autonomic involvement (eg, cardiac irregularities, hypertension, or hypotension) may be severe
  - Electromyography consistent with demyelinating injury
  - Lumbar puncture, normal in early or mild disease, shows high protein, normal cell count
  - Associated with viral infections, inoculation, stress, and preceding *Campylobacter jejuni* enteritis, but most cases do not have any definitive link to pathogens

- ■ Differential Diagnosis
  - Diphtheria, poliomyelitis (where endemic)
  - Porphyria
  - Heavy metal poisoning
  - Botulism
  - Transverse myelitis of any origin

- ■ Treatment
  - Pulmonary functions closely monitored, with intubation for forced vital capacity < 15 mL/kg
  - Respiratory and physical therapy
  - Plasmapheresis or intravenous immunoglobulin for clinically severe or rapidly progressive cases
  - Up to 20% of patients are left with persisting disability

12

Bell's Palsy (Idiopathic Facial Paresis)

- **Essentials of Diagnosis**   CN VII
  - An idiopathic facial paresis of the lower motor neuron type
  - Abrupt onset of hemifacial (including the forehead) weakness, difficulty closing eye; ipsilateral ear pain may precede or accompany weakness
  - Unilateral peripheral seventh nerve palsy on examination; taste preserved on posterior tongue

- **Differential Diagnosis**
  - Cerebrovascular accident
  - Intracranial mass lesion
  - Basilar meningitis, especially that associated with sarcoidosis

- **Treatment**
  - Supportive measures with frequent eye lubrication and nocturnal eye patching
  - Corticosteroid management controversial; may be indicated when palsy is complete or pain present
  - Only 10% of patients are dissatisfied with the final outcome of their disability or disfigurement

12

Combined System Disease
(Posterolateral Sclerosis)

■ Essentials of Diagnosis

- Numbness ("pins and needles"); tenderness; weakness; feeling of heaviness in toes, feet, fingers, and hands
- Stocking and glove distribution of sensory loss in some patients
- Extensor plantar response and hyperreflexia typical, as is loss of position and vibratory sense
- Serum vitamin B_{12} level low
- Megaloblastic anemia may be present but does not parallel neurologic dysfunction

■ Differential Diagnosis

- Tabes dorsalis
- Multiple sclerosis
- Transverse myelitis of viral origin
- Epidural tumor or abscess
- Cervical spondylosis

■ Treatment

- Vitamin B_{12}

12

Myasthenia Gravis

- ■ Essentials of Diagnosis
  - Symptoms due to a variable degree of block of neuromuscular transmission
  - Fluctuating weakness of musculature with characteristic worsening with repetitive use; diplopia, dysphagia, ptosis, facial weakness, especially with chewing and speaking
  - Short-acting anticholinesterases transiently increase strength
  - Electromyography and nerve conduction studies demonstrate decremental muscle response to repeated stimuli
  - Associations include thymic tumors, thyrotoxicosis, rheumatoid arthritis, and SLE
  - Elevated acetylcholine receptor antibody assay confirmatory

- ■ Differential Diagnosis
  - Polyneuropathy due to other causes
  - Amyotrophic lateral sclerosis
  - Botulism
  - Bulbar poliomyelitis
  - Neuromuscular blocking drug toxicity (aminoglycosides)
  - Primary myopathy, eg, polymyositis
  - Lambert-Eaton syndrome

12

- ■ Treatment
  - Anticholinesterase drugs, particularly pyridostigmine, may be effective
  - Thymectomy if patient under age 60 and otherwise healthy and weakness not restricted to extraocular muscles
  - Corticosteroids and immunosuppressants if response to anticholinesterase drugs and thymectomy poor
  - Plasmapheresis or intravenous immunoglobulin therapy provides short-term benefit in selected patients
  - Avoid aminoglycosides, which may exacerbate disease

Periodic Paralysis Syndromes

- ■ Essentials of Diagnosis
  - Episodes of flaccid weakness or paralysis with strength normal between attacks
  - Hypokalemic variety: attacks may be prolonged upon awakening, after exercise or after carbohydrate meals; hyperthyroidism commonly associated in Asian males
  - Hyperkalemic variety or normokalemic variety: brief attacks post exercise

- ■ Differential Diagnosis
  - Myasthenia gravis
  - Polyneuropathies, especially Guillain-Barré syndrome
  - Posterior circulation stroke
  - Primary myopathy of other cause

- ■ Treatment
  - Hypokalemic variant: potassium replacement for acute episode; low-carbohydrate, low-salt diet chronically, perhaps acetazolamide prophylactically; treatment of hyperthyroidism, when associated, reduces attacks, as does therapy with beta-blockers
  - Hyper/normokalemic variant: intravenous calcium, intravenous diuretics useful for acute therapy; prophylactic acetazolamide or thiazides also beneficial

12

Trigeminal Neuralgia (Tic Douloureux)

- ■ Essentials of Diagnosis
    - • Characterized by momentary episodes of lancinating facial pain that arises from one side of the mouth and shoots toward the ipsilateral eye, ear, or nostril
    - • Commonly affects women more than men in middle and later life
    - • Triggered by touch, movement, drafts, and eating
    - • Symptoms are confined to the distribution of the ipsilateral trigeminal nerve (usually the second or third division)
    - • Occasionally caused by multiple sclerosis or a brainstem tumor

- ■ Differential Diagnosis
    - • Atypical facial pain syndrome
    - • Glossopharyngeal neuralgia
    - • Postherpetic neuralgia
    - • Temporomandibular joint dysfunction
    - • Angina pectoris

- ■ Treatment
    - • Carbamazepine is usually the drug of choice; if this is ineffective or poorly tolerated, phenytoin or baclofen can be tried
    - • Surgical exploration of posterior fossa successful in selected patients

12

13

Psychiatric Disorders

Delirium, Dementia, & Other Cognitive Disorders

- **Essentials of Diagnosis**
  - Transient or permanent cognitive impairment
  - Emotional disorders including depression, anxiety, or irritability frequently present
  - Behavioral disturbance with decreased impulse control, attention deficits, aggression, exhibitionism or sexual acting-out
  - Numerous causes include intoxications, drug withdrawal, alcoholism, infection, hypoxia, endocrinopathies, central nervous system neoplasm, fluid and electrolyte disturbances, nutritional deficiency, trauma, seizures, autoimmune disorders, degenerative diseases (eg, Alzheimer's disease), and medications

- **Differential Diagnosis**
  - Functional psychoses
  - Primary dementia or pseudodementia

- **Treatment**
  - Identify and treat underlying cause if reversible
  - Stabilize living environment
  - Behavioral or social therapy

Anxiety Disorders (Neuroses)

- ■ Essentials of Diagnosis
  - Includes generalized anxiety disorder, panic disorder, obsessive-compulsive disorder, dissociative disorder (eg, fugue, amnesia, multiple personality), and phobic disorder; occasionally difficult to diagnose, especially panic disorder
  - Overt anxiety or overt manifestation of a defense mechanism (eg, phobia)
  - Tension, fears, difficulty in concentration, apprehension
  - No situational basis for symptoms
  - Somatic symptoms referable to autonomic nervous system or specific organ system (eg, dyspnea, palpitations, paresthesias)
  - Not a result of physical disorders, psychiatric conditions (eg, schizophrenia), or stimulant drugs (eg, cocaine or caffeine)

- ■ Differential Diagnosis
  - Endocrinopathies (eg, thyrotoxicosis)
  - Alcohol withdrawal
  - Pheochromocytoma
  - Substance abuse

- ■ Treatment
  - Avoidance of stimulants
  - Generalized anxiety disorder: behavioral therapy plus medication in short courses (benzodiazepines and buspirone are the drugs of choice); beta-blockers for symptomatic relief
  - Panic disorder: behavioral or cognitive therapy plus medication (selective serotonin reuptake inhibitors or monoamine oxidase inhibitors)
  - Obsessive-compulsive disorder: behavioral or cognitive therapy plus medication (selective serotonin reuptake inhibitors)

13

Somatoform Disorders (Psychosomatic Disorders)

- ■ Essentials of Diagnosis
  - Includes conversion, somatization, pain disorder with psychologic features, hypochondriasis, and factitious illness
  - Symptoms may involve one or more organ systems and are unintentional
  - Subjective complaints exceed objective findings
  - Symptom development correlates with psychosocial stress

- ■ Differential Diagnosis
  - Major depression
  - Anatomic disease of organ system producing symptoms

- ■ Treatment
  - Attention to building therapeutic doctor-patient relationship
  - Acknowledgment that patient's distress is real
  - Psychotherapy
  - Behavioral modification
  - Biofeedback; hypnosis

13

Chronic Pain Disorders

- ■ Essentials of Diagnosis
  - Chronic complaints of pain
  - Symptoms exceed objective signs
  - Minimal relief with standard therapies
  - History of multiple physician consultations common
  - Frequent use of polypharmacy

- ■ Differential Diagnosis
  - Depression
  - Anxiety disorder
  - Superimposed organic or structural disease involving painful areas
  - Somatoform disorder

- ■ Treatment
  - One physician should assume responsibility for care of patient
  - Comprehensive behavioral approach (eg, biofeedback, hypnosis, behavioral modification)
  - Fixed schedule of analgesic medication (as opposed to "as needed")
  - Make the patient a partner in treatment efforts; formal medication contracts often helpful
  - Group therapy with family and other patients

13

Personality Disorders

- ■ Essentials of Diagnosis
  - Includes paranoid, schizoid, compulsive, histrionic, schizotypal, narcissistic, avoidant, dependent, passive-aggressive, antisocial, and borderline personality disorders
  - History dating to childhood of recurrent maladaptive behavior, low self-esteem, and lack of confidence
  - Minimal introspective ability
  - Major, recurrent difficulties with interpersonal relationships
  - Depression with anxiety when maladaptive behavior fails

- ■ Differential Diagnosis
  - Anxiety
  - Dissociative disorder
  - Depression
  - Psychotic disorder

- ■ Treatment
  - Maintenance of a highly structured environment
  - Behavioral therapy with operant and aversive conditioning
  - Group therapy
  - Antipsychotic medications (haloperidol) may be required transiently

13

Psychotic Disorders

- ■ Essentials of Diagnosis
    - This group of disorders includes schizophrenia, paranoid disorder, schizoaffective and schizophreniform disorder, brief reactive psychosis, late life psychosis, and atypical psychosis
    - Social withdrawal, often progressive; deterioration of personal care, loss of ego boundaries; loose thought associations
    - Autistic absorption in inner thoughts and frequent sexual or religious preoccupations
    - Auditory hallucinations, delusions, flat or inappropriate affect
    - Concrete thinking with inability to abstract; impaired concentration; depersonalization
    - Symptoms of at least 6 months' duration

- ■ Differential Diagnosis
    - Atypical affective disorder
    - Mania
    - Reactive psychosis
    - Drug toxicity
    - Psychotic depression
    - Seizure disorder
    - Endocrinopathies (eg, thyrotoxicosis)

- ■ Treatment
    - High-potency antipsychotic medications (eg, phenothiazines)
    - Attempt to stabilize living situation
    - Psychotherapy may be effective for previously adjusted patients with a single psychotic episode
    - Behavioral therapy

13

Affective Disorders (Depression & Mania)

- ■ Essentials of Diagnosis
  - Includes adjustment disorder with depressed mood, major depression, dysthymia, depression not otherwise specified, mania, cyclothymic disorder, and mood disorder secondary to illness and drugs
  - Altered mood with intense feelings of sadness, guilt, worthlessness, and hopelessness
  - Poor concentration, anhedonia, somatic complaints such as headache, altered sleep or appetite pattern, decreased sexual drive
  - Psychomotor retardation, inability to concentrate, difficulty thinking
  - In patients with bipolar disorder, depression may alternate with periods of mania (hyperactivity, racing thoughts, grandiosity, sleep disruption, euphoria, irritability)

- ■ Differential Diagnosis
  - Depression due to any medical illness or drug toxicity
  - Mania due to thyrotoxicosis or drug toxicity

- ■ Treatment
  - Assess suicidal risk in all patients; hospitalize patients who are suicidal
  - Psychotherapy, social therapy, behavioral therapy, or pharmacotherapy (eg, tricyclic antidepressants, selective serotonin reuptake inhibitors, trazodone, bupropion) for depression
  - Electroconvulsive therapy for refractory cases of depression
  - Haloperidol for acute manic episodes with lithium for long-term management
  - Carbamazepine and valproic acid also effective in patients with mania
  - Psychotherapy or social and behavioral modification may be of value once acute manic episode is controlled

13

Alcoholism

- ■ Essentials of Diagnosis
  - • Physiologic dependence with symptoms of withdrawal when intake is interrupted
  - • Tolerance to the effects of alcohol
  - • Presence of alcohol-associated medical illnesses (eg, liver disease, cerebellar degeneration)
  - • Continued drinking despite strong medical and social contraindications and life disruptions
  - • Impairment in social and occupational functioning
  - • Depression

- ■ Differential Diagnosis
  - • Alcohol abuse secondary to underlying major psychiatric illness
  - • In withdrawal states, must exclude other sedative or drug toxicities, organic brain syndromes, and medical illnesses

- ■ Treatment
  - • Address the problem of denial with patient and family members
  - • Total abstinence, not "controlled drinking," should be the goal
  - • Social therapy (eg, Alcoholics Anonymous)
  - • Disulfiram in selected patients; naltrexone may also prove to be of benefit
  - • Benzodiazepines, clonidine, or propranolol for withdrawal symptoms
  - • Haloperidol for hallucinations
  - • Treat underlying psychiatric illness if present

13

Opioid Dependency

- **Essentials of Diagnosis**
  - Intoxication: Somnolence, slurred speech, ataxia, coma, respiratory depression, miotic pupils
  - Physical dependence with tolerance and extreme motivation to obtain illicit drugs
  - Withdrawal uncomfortable but not life-threatening

- **Differential Diagnosis**
  - Alcoholism or other sedative dependency (may be related)
  - Encephalitis
  - Metabolic encephalopathy, eg, hypercapnia, hypoxia, hypoglycemia

- **Treatment**
  - Naloxone for suspected overdose with close medical observation
  - Methadone maintenance after withdrawal for selected patients
  - Clonidine may be helpful in alleviating the cardiovascular symptoms of withdrawal
  - Psychotherapy, social and behavioral therapy, or group therapy may be helpful

13

Sedative or Hypnotic Dependency

- ■ Essentials of Diagnosis
  - Intoxication: confusion, slurred speech, somnolence, ataxia, coma, respiratory depression
  - History often unreliable or unobtainable; high index of suspicion necessary
  - Euphoria, excitement, aggressive behavior paradoxically found in elderly
  - Tolerance with psychologic and physical dependence

- ■ Differential Diagnosis
  - Alcoholism
  - Other acute intoxications
  - Psychosis of functional origin
  - Coma due to metabolic disturbance or structural disease

- ■ Treatment
  - As in all overdoses, gastric lavage and activated charcoal with medical support
  - Address reasons for dependency with short-term psychotherapy
  - Social and behavioral therapy, group therapy may help

13

14

Dermatologic Disorders

Vascular Birthmarks

- ■ Essentials of Diagnosis
  - Macular or papular lesion varying in color but usually red or bluish

- ■ Differential Diagnosis
  - Port wine stain
  - Strawberry hemangioma
  - Lymphangioma

- ■ Treatment
  - Reassure parents that most vascular birthmarks regress
  - Surgical treatment for selected cases
  - Laser coagulation of selected birthmarks

Contact Dermatitis (Dermatitis Venenata)

- ■ Essentials of Diagnosis
  - • Pruritus, burning, and stinging, often intense
  - • Erythema and edema often, in many cases followed by vesicles and bullae in area of contact with suspected agent
  - • Later: weeping, crusting, and sometimes secondary infection
  - • Eruption confined to region of direct skin contact with allergen and may suggest etiologic agent (eg, jewelry, fingernail polish)
  - • Usually asymmetric distribution of eruption, except when associated with apparel
  - • Often a history of previous reaction to suspected contactant
  - • Patch test with agent usually positive in the allergic form

- ■ Differential Diagnosis
  - • Atopic dermatitis or other eczemas
  - • Scabies
  - • Dermatophytoses
  - • Herpes simplex if lesions vesicular
  - • Impetigo

- ■ Treatment
  - • Prevent reexposure to causative agents; increasing sensitivity to occupational agents may necessitate change of work exposure
  - • Topical symptomatic treatment with steroid creams or soothing formulations
  - • Short courses of oral corticosteroids (prednisone, 40–60 mg/d tapered over 2–3 weeks) for severe cases
  - • Treatment of secondary bacterial or fungal infections, if present

14

Erythema Nodosum

- ■ Essentials of Diagnosis
  - Women predominantly affected
  - Painful red nodules, usually over anterior aspect of legs
  - Absence of ulceration
  - Systemic signs and symptoms, including fever, chills, malaise, headache, or myalgia, may be present; additional signs and symptoms may be manifestation of an underlying cause
  - Slow regression over several weeks to resemble contusions
  - Most cases associated with infection, drug sensitivity (penicillin, progestins), or underlying systemic disease (ulcerative colitis, sarcoidosis, leukemia)
  - Laboratory tests should be dictated by suspected underlying causes: serologic tests depending upon history of possible exposure to *Coccidioides immitis,* streptococcus, syphilis, various fungi, or hepatitis B may be indicated.
  - Appropriate investigation if inflammatory bowel disease, *Yersinia* infection, or *Salmonella* infection suspected

- ■ Differential Diagnosis
  - Resolving bruises
  - Thrombophlebitis
  - Erythema chronicum migrans (Lyme disease)
  - Nodular vasculitis
  - Erythema induratum
  - Erythema multiforme
  - Lupus panniculitis

- ■ Treatment
  - Identify and treat underlying cause if present
  - Bed rest with legs slightly elevated while pain is severe
  - NSAIDs
  - Steroids only for severely symptomatic patients
  - Potassium iodide orally may provide prompt regression, but efficacy and safety unclear

14

Erythema Multiforme

- **Essentials of Diagnosis**
  - Sudden onset of symmetric erythematous skin lesions with history of recurrence
  - May be macular, papular, urticarial, bullous, or purpuric
  - "Target" lesions with clear centers and concentric erythematous rings may be noted
  - Predilection for extensor surfaces, palms, soles, or mucous membranes
  - Associated conditions include herpes simplex, systemic infection, or drugs (eg, sulfonamides)
  - Stevens-Johnson syndrome, a dermatologic emergency, is a serious variant usually involving two mucous membranes (often oral and conjunctival), including the tracheobronchial tree
  - Laboratory evaluations should include serologic tests for syphilis and skin biopsy, which may demonstrate herpes virus antigen as causative agent and is helpful to distinguish erythema multiforme from variants of urticaria

- **Differential Diagnosis**
  - Fixed drug eruption
  - Urticarial papules may resemble urticaria or insect bites
  - Secondary syphilis may be mistaken for palm and sole involvement
  - Bullous changes similar to dermatitis herpetiformis, pemphigus, toxic epidermal necrolysis

- **Treatment**
  - Identify underlying cause
  - Specific therapy should be aimed at discontinuing offending drugs or treating underlying infection if present
  - Stevens-Johnson variant is best treated as burn; corticosteroids are usually given

14

Pemphigus

■ Essentials of Diagnosis

- Relapsing crops of flaccid bullae appearing on normal skin
- Often preceded by mucous membrane bullae, erosions, and ulcerations
- Superficial detachment of skin after lateral traction (Nikolsky's sign) often present
- Cause unknown, but may be associated with other autoimmune diseases such as myasthenia gravis, lupus erythematosus, thymoma, or bullous pemphigoid
- May be precipitated by captopril or penicillamine
- Smear taken from base of bullae and stained with Giemsa's stain demonstrates disruption of epidermal intercellular connections (acantholysis)
- Intercellular antibody may be detected by indirect immunofluorescence of patient's serum

■ Differential Diagnosis

(***Note:*** Acantholysis not a feature of these other conditions.)
- Erythema multiforme
- Dermatitis herpetiformis
- Drug eruption
- Contact dermatitis
- Bullous impetigo
- Pemphigoid

■ Treatment

- Supportive care and rest
- High-dose corticosteroids (180–360 mg/d for 6–10 weeks)
- Tetracycline and nicotinamide may also be useful in patients with stable disease
- Antimetabolites and alkylating agents for selected severe cases
- Meticulous care of denuded skin to prevent infection
- Complicating infection requires appropriate antibiotic therapy

14

Atopic Dermatitis (Eczema)

- **Essentials of Diagnosis**
  - Pruritic, exudative, or lichenified eruption with predilection for face, neck, upper truck, wrists, hands, and folds of knees and elbows
  - Personal or family history of atopy (eg, asthma, allergic rhinitis, or eczema)
  - Tendency to recur after remissions from adolescence to young adulthood
  - Laboratory tests may reveal eosinophilia and radioimmunologic allergen-specific IgE

- **Differential Diagnosis**
  - Seborrheic dermatitis
  - Contact dermatitis
  - Lichen simplex chronicus
  - Impetigo

- **Treatment**
  - Treat symptomatically depending upon stage of lesion; acute lesions managed with soothing soaks, whereas chronic lesions best treated with ointments, topical steroids, and tar preparations.
  - Topical corticosteroids may be used sparingly; brief courses of systemic steroids should be used only in highly selected cases
  - Antihistamines to relieve pruritus
  - Dietary measures and desensitization are of limited value
  - Treat complicating staphylococcal infections with systemic antibiotics

14

Lichen Simplex Chronicus
(Localized Neurodermatitis)

- **Essentials of Diagnosis**
  - Chronic pruritus and scratching associated with pigmented lichenified skin lesions
  - Exaggerated skin lines overlying a thickened, well-circumscribed scaly plaque
  - Predilection for nape of neck, wrists, external surfaces of forearms, inner thighs, genitalia, posterior popliteal and antecubital areas
  - Affected areas in reach of patient's fingers
  - Said to be related to stress

- **Differential Diagnosis**
  - Atopic dermatitis
  - Seborrheic dermatitis
  - Psoriasis
  - Lichen planus
  - Mycosis fungoides
  - Lichenoid drug eruption

- **Treatment**
  - Cover affected area
  - Topical or intralesional steroids
  - Anxiolytics may be helpful
  - Stress reduction measures

14

Dermatitis Medicamentosa (Drug Eruption)

- **Essentials of Diagnosis**
  - Usually abrupt onset of widespread, symmetric erythematous eruption, mimicking any inflammatory condition
  - Constitutional symptoms (malaise, arthralgia, headache, and fever) may be present
  - Direct immunofluorescence studies positive for some drugs (eg, sulfonamides, NSAIDs) to distinguish them from other eruptions

- **Differential Diagnosis**
  - Distinguished from other eruptions by history and resolution following drug withdrawal

- **Treatment**
  - Discontinue all drugs if possible
  - Antihistamines, epinephrine, and corticosteroids for urticarial or anaphylactoid manifestations
  - Treat local eruptions symptomatically

Exfoliative Dermatitis (Exfoliative Erythroderma)

- **Essentials of Diagnosis**
  - Scaling and erythema involving large area of body
  - Pruritus, malaise, fever, weight loss
  - Primary disease or exposure to toxic agent (contact, oral, parenteral) may be evident
  - Causative factors include preexisting dermatosis (psoriasis, atopic dermatitis, etc), exposure to toxin, underlying malignancy (10%); or may be idiopathic

- **Differential Diagnosis**
  (*Note:* Any of the following may themselves become exfoliative.)
  - Severe psoriasis
  - Lichen planus
  - Extensive seborrheic dermatitis
  - Dermatitis medicamentosa

- **Treatment**
  - Discontinue all drugs if possible
  - Bed rest with talc on bedsheets
  - Short-term corticosteroids for severe exfoliation
  - Local skin care for less severe presentations

14

Photodermatitis

- ■ Essentials of Diagnosis
  - Painful erythema, edema, and vesiculation on sun-exposed surfaces
  - Fever, gastrointestinal symptoms, malaise, or prostration may occur
  - Proteinuria, casts, and hematuria may occur
  - Porphyrins may be measured to rule out porphyria

- ■ Differential Diagnosis
  - Contact dermatitis from sunscreen
  - Lupus erythematosus
  - Porphyrias
  - Polymorphous light eruption

- ■ Treatment
  - Discontinue potentially photosensitizing drugs
  - Avoidance of prolonged exposure to ultraviolet radiation and use of sunscreens when exposed to sunlight
  - Soothing local measures as for any acute dermatitis
  - Chloroquine for associated porphyria cutanea tarda may be useful

Lichen Planus

- ## Essentials of Diagnosis
  - Pruritic, violaceous, flat-topped papules with fine white streaks and symmetric distribution
  - Predilection for anterior wrists, sacral region, penis, legs, and mucous membranes
  - Commonly seen along areas of linear trauma (Köbner's phenomenon)
  - Histopathology is diagnostic, revealing band infiltration of T cells in dermis; immunofluorescent demonstration of C3 and IgG at basement membrane
  - Usually occurs in an otherwise healthy but anxious individual; more common in females

- ## Differential Diagnosis
  - Psoriasis
  - Papular eczema
  - Syphilis
  - Leukoplakia, if on mucous membranes
  - Chemical sensitivity, including bismuth, quinacrine, and photographic developing solutions

- ## Treatment
  - Anxiolytic agents
  - Corticosteroids systemically or intralesionally may be helpful for severe cases
  - Use of retinoids, topically or systemically, is controversial

14

Psoriasis

- ■ Essentials of Diagnosis
  - Silvery scales on bright red plaques with predilection for knees, elbows, and scalp
  - Nail pitting
  - Pruritus is mild unless psoriasis is eruptive or occurs in body folds
  - Psoriatic arthritis (distal interphalangeal joints, other peripheral joints, spondylitis) may be an associated manifestation
  - Extensive erythrodermic psoriasis of abrupt onset may accompany AIDS
  - Histopathologic features are specific

- ■ Differential Diagnosis
  - Seborrheic dermatitis
  - Candidal intertrigo
  - Onychomycosis
  - Reiter's syndrome

- ■ Treatment
  - Apply lotions containing coal tar to affected area; alternatively, fluorinated corticosteroids applied overnight under occlusive plastic wrapping
  - Daily warm baths with scrubbing of lesions for more chronic affliction
  - Combination of ultraviolet irradiations and coal tar (variation of Goeckerman regimen) for long-standing and severe lesions
  - Psoralen plus ultraviolet-A light (PUVA) is used in refractory cases
  - Systemic retinoids are first choice for severe pustular psoriasis and may be helpful for psoriatic arthritis; methotrexate valuable in this situation as well

14

Pityriasis Rosea

- ■ Essentials of Diagnosis
    - Oval, fawn-colored, scaly eruption following the cleavage lines of the trunk in a Christmas tree distribution
    - Herald patch commonly precedes eruption by 1–2 weeks
    - Occasional pruritus

- ■ Differential Diagnosis
    - Secondary syphilis
    - Seborrheic dermatitis
    - Truncal fungal infections
    - Drug eruption
    - Guttate psoriasis
    - Erythema chronicum migrans

- ■ Treatment
    - Reassurance is sufficient in most cases, since there is spontaneous remission in 6–12 weeks

14

Seborrheic Dermatitis & Dandruff

- **Essentials of Diagnosis**
  - Dry scales or dry yellowish dandruff with or without underlying erythema
  - Scalp, central face, presternal, interscapular areas, umbilicus, and body folds may be involved
  - Patients with Parkinson's disease develop severe seborrheic dermatitis
  - Overgrowth of *Pityrosporum ovale* involved with seborrheic dermatitis in AIDS patients

- **Differential Diagnosis**
  - Intertrigo
  - Fungal infections
  - Psoriasis

- **Treatment**
  - Selenium sulfide shampoo
  - Corticosteroid creams and lotions
  - Oral ketoconazole for severe cases
  - Ketoconazole 2% cream to treat *P ovalis* in AIDS patients

Acne Vulgaris

- ■ Essentials of Diagnosis
  - Papules or pustules over the face, back, and shoulders, with onset at puberty and often persisting into adulthood
  - Open and closed comedones
  - Cyst formation, slow resolution, scarring
  - Consider hyperandrogenism when resistant case encountered in a woman

- ■ Differential Diagnosis
  - Halide toxicity
  - Contact dermatitis caused by naphthalenes
  - Excess of glucocorticosteroids
  - Tuberous sclerosis
  - Molluscum contagiosum

- ■ Treatment
  - Antibiotics such as tetracycline, erythromycin, or minocycline are very effective; occasionally, topical erythromycin or clindamycin is useful
  - Topical keratolytic agents such as tretinoin
  - Intralesional steroids for cysts
  - Oral contraceptives occasionally for young women to counter hyperandrogenism
  - Oral retinoids for the most severe cases only (absolutely contraindicated in pregnancy due to teratogenicity)
  - Dermabrasion for cosmetic improvement of superficial scars

14

Rosacea

- ■ **Essentials of Diagnosis**
    - A chronic facial disorder of middle-aged and elderly individuals
    - Erythema and telangiectasis are prominent
    - An acneiform component (papules, pustules, and seborrhea) is present
    - Hyperplasia of the soft tissue of the nose (rhinophyma) observed in many patients
    - Emotional disturbances, migraine headaches, chronic alcoholism, underlying seborrhea, and gastrointestinal tract disturbances are associated factors in some patients

- ■ **Differential Diagnosis**
    - Acne vulgaris
    - Halide toxicity
    - Demodicidosis (mite *Demodex folliculorum* found in pores)
    - SLE
    - Carcinoid syndrome

- ■ **Treatment**
    - Elimination of alcohol
    - Oral tetracycline
    - Low-dose retinoids
    - Topical steroids
    - Rhinophyma may be treated surgically in selected patients

14

Urticaria & Angioedema

- ■ Essentials of Diagnosis
  - Pruritic eruptions of evanescent wheals or hives of heterogeneous origins involving lips, tongue, eyelids, larynx, palms, soles, or genitalia
  - Special forms have characteristic features (hereditary angio-edema, dermatographism, cholinergic urticaria, solar urticaria, cold urticaria)
  - Most episodes are acute and self-limited over a period of 1–2 weeks
  - Chronic urticaria patients should be evaluated for underlying systemic illness such as vasculitis, lymphoma, or hepatitis B

- ■ Differential Diagnosis
  - Unmistakable; only question is particular cause

- ■ Treatment
  - Eliminate underlying cause if identifiable
  - Antihistamines are mainstay for allergic urticaria
  - Short courses of steroids and sometimes epinephrine may be necessary for severe manifestations
  - Androgens (danazol or stanozolol) for hereditary angioedema
  - H_2 blockers in conjunction with H_1 blockers used with inconsistent results for chronic urticaria

14

Miliaria (Heat Rash)

- ■ Essentials of Diagnosis
    - • An acute dermatitis usually occurring on the upper extremities, trunk, and intertriginous areas
    - • Burning and pruritus; superficial aggregated small vesicles, papules, or pustules on covered areas of skin
    - • Usually occurs in hot, moist climate
    - • May have fever and even heat prostration with severe forms that interfere with heat regulation

- ■ Differential Diagnosis
    - • Drug allergy
    - • Folliculitis

- ■ Treatment
    - • Antipruritic cooling lotion containing a steroid, phenol, and menthol is effective
    - • Antibiotics for secondary superficial pyoderma
    - • Avoidance of environmental predisposing factors
    - • Oral anticholinergic medications for severe cases

14

Anogenital Pruritus

- ■ Essentials of Diagnosis
  - Pruritus, chiefly nocturnal, of the anogenital area
  - There may be no skin reactions, but inflammation of any degree up to lichenification may occur
  - Multiple specific causes may include oxyuriasis (pinworm), irritants, diabetes, or fungal infection, but usually no specific cause is identified
  - Laboratory studies to evaluate diabetes; microscopic scrapings for fungi or parasites may be useful

- ■ Differential Diagnosis
  - Candidiasis
  - Psoriasis
  - Seborrheic dermatitis

- ■ Treatment
  - Proper anogenital hygiene
  - Avoid spicy foods that may irritate anal mucosa
  - Psyllium laxatives for associated constipation
  - Local hydrocortisone
  - Sitz baths with topical astringents for inflammation

14

Chronic Discoid Lupus Erythematosus

- **Essentials of Diagnosis**
  - Red, asymptomatic, localized plaques, usually on the face, often in butterfly distribution
  - Scaling, follicular plugging, atrophy, and telangiectasia of involved areas that may result in depigmentation and scarring
  - Histologic features are distinctive, revealing basement membrane antibody in involved areas of skin
  - May be photosensitive
  - ANA often positive, but dsDNA antibody studies negative

- **Differential Diagnosis**
  - Seborrheic dermatitis
  - Basal cell epithelioma
  - Lupus vulgaris
  - Rosacea

- **Treatment**
  - Avoidance of sunlight and any form of radiation therapy
  - Intralesional or topical steroid therapy should be attempted initially
  - Antimalarials (with periodic ophthalmologic examinations) for more severe cases

Herpes Simplex

- ■ Essentials of Diagnosis
    - Recurrent small grouped vesicles on an erythematous base, especially involving oral and genital areas
    - Burning and stinging are predominant symptoms
    - May follow minor infections, trauma, stress, or sun exposure
    - Regional lymphadenopathy, especially in primary infection
    - Tzanck smear (obtained from base of vesicle) positive for large multinucleated epithelial giant cells surrounded by acantholytic balloon cells
    - Immunofluorescence techniques to detect viral antigen

- ■ Differential Diagnosis
    - Impetigo
    - Sexually transmitted diseases, including syphilis, chancroid, and lymphogranuloma venereum

- ■ Treatment
    - Systemic oral acyclovir (200 mg five times daily for 10 days) decreases symptoms and shortens course of herpes infection; topical zinc sulfate in camphor water also useful in immunocompetent patients
    - Intravenous acyclovir effective but has little role in local disease and is reserved for life-threatening manifestations
    - Topical acyclovir for first episode of genital herpes and mucocutaneous herpes in immunocompromised patients

14

Herpes Zoster (Shingles)

- ■ Essentials of Diagnosis
  - Pain along course of a nerve followed by eruption of painful grouped vesicular lesions
  - Etiologic agent is morphologically identical to varicella virus
  - Unilateral involvement with predilection for face and trunk
  - Swelling of regional lymph nodes is inconsistent finding
  - Dissemination may occur in immunocompromised individuals
  - Severe initial pain in patients over 50–60 years of age increases likelihood of postherpetic neuralgia
  - Ocular involvement may be severe with V_1 distribution of lesions, predicted by lesion on tip of nose
  - Tzanck smear obtained from base of vesicle is positive

- ■ Differential Diagnosis
  - Contact dermatitis
  - Visceral diseases associated with pain in the same distribution, including myocardial infarction, cholecystitis, or migraine, may be confused with preeruptive shingles

- ■ Treatment
  - Intravenous or high-dose oral acyclovir (800 mg orally daily for 7 days) accelerates healing and ameliorates symptoms
  - Administrations of short courses of prednisone in high doses for patients over 50 years of age is controversial but may decrease the incidence of postherpetic neuralgia
  - Prompt ophthalmologic consultation if there is involvement of the first branch of the trigeminal nerve
  - Calamine lotion or starch shake lotions may be useful
  - Topical capsaicin, regional nerve blocks, and antidepressants appear to help some patients with postherpetic neuralgia

14

Verruca Vulgaris (Warts)

- ■ Essentials of Diagnosis
  - Warty elevation anywhere on skin or mucous membranes, usually no larger than 0.5 cm in diameter
  - Etiologic agent is human papillomavirus
  - Prolonged incubation period (average 2–18 months)
  - Spontaneous "cures" frequent (50%), but lesions often unresponsive to any form of treatment
  - "Recurrences" (new lesions) are frequent

- ■ Differential Diagnosis
  - Basal cell epitheliomas

- ■ Treatment
  - Avoid contact with warts
  - Surgical excision
  - Removal using liquid nitrogen
  - Keratolytic agents
  - Podophyllum resin for anogenital warts
  - Salicylic acid 40% plaster application after paring for plantar warts

14

Folliculitis

- ■ Essentials of Diagnosis
  - Pruritus and burning in areas containing hair follicles
  - Pustules in the hair follicles usually caused by staphylococcal infection
  - Inflammation of surrounding skin in selected cases
  - "Hot tub folliculitis" caused by *Pseudomonas aeruginosa* characterized by pruritic truncal rash occurring 1–4 days after bathing in hot tub, swimming pool, or whirlpool
  - Pseudofolliculitis caused by ingrowing hairs in beard area treated by growing beard or using depilatory

- ■ Differential Diagnosis
  - Acne vulgaris
  - Localized fungal infections
  - Impetigo
  - Pustular miliaria

- ■ Treatment
  - Local antibiotic or chlorhexidine
  - Systemic antimicrobials if above measures fail or if disease severe or involving upper lip or nose, which is associated with the rare complication of cavernous sinus thrombosis
  - Anhydrous ethyl alcohol containing 6.25% aluminum chloride applied to lesions followed by antibiotic ointment especially useful for chronic folliculitis of the buttocks

14

Furuncles (Boils) & Carbuncles

- **Essentials of Diagnosis**
  - Furuncle: a painful, inflammatory swelling of a hair follicle and adjacent subcutaneous tissue forming an abscess
  - Coagulase-positive *Staphylococcus aureus* is the causative organism
  - Carbuncle: composed of multiple furuncles coalescing and forming a deep abscess with multiple drainage points
  - Primary predisposing disease sometimes present, eg, diabetes mellitus
  - Sites of occurrence are hairy parts exposed to irritation, pressure, or moisture

- **Differential Diagnosis**
  - Deep fungal infections (sporotrichosis and blastomycosis)
  - Anthrax
  - Tularemia
  - Cystic acne
  - Infected epidermal cysts
  - Hidradenitis suppuritiva

- **Treatment**
  - Systemic antistaphylococcal antibiotics such as sodium dicloxacillin, erythromycin, or cephalexin
  - Avoidance of manipulation of inflamed areas
  - Incision and drainage after lesions are well demarcated

14

Erysipelas

- **Essentials of Diagnosis**
  - A superficial form of cellulitis, occurring classically on the cheek, caused by beta-hemolytic streptococci
  - Edematous, spreading, sharply demarcated, hot, erythematous area, with or without vesicle or bulla formation characterized by spreading margin
  - Pain, malaise, chills and fever
  - Blood cultures may be positive

- **Differential Diagnosis**
  - Cellulitis
  - Erysipeloid

- **Treatment**
  - Intravenous penicillin or erythromycin
  - Bed rest with head elevation

14

Tinea Capitis (Ringworm of Scalp)

- ■ Essentials of Diagnosis
    - Round, gray, scaly "bald" patches on scalp
    - Usually noted in children between ages 2 and 6 years
    - Lymphadenitis may occur even with subtle scalp disease
    - Occasionally fluorescent under Wood's lamp
    - Microscopic examination or culture identifies *Microsporum* or *Trichophyton* fungal organisms

- ■ Differential Diagnosis
    - Alopecia areata
    - Trichotillomania
    - Pediculosis pyoderma
    - Seborrheic dermatitis (very uncommon in children 2–8 years of age)
    - Impetigo

- ■ Treatment
    - Avoid sharing headgear with infected individuals
    - Microcrystalline griseofulvin orally for 8 weeks
    - Selenium sulfide shampoo to reduce spore shedding

14

Tinea Corporis or Tinea Circinata (Body Ringworm)

- ■ Essentials of Diagnosis
  - Intensely pruritic, ringed, scaling, centrally clearing lesions; small vesicles in a peripherally advancing border
  - Predilection for exposed skin surfaces
  - May be caused by all species of dermatophytes
  - History of exposure to infected domestic animal
  - Examination of scrapings in 10% potassium hydroxide demonstrates hyphae
  - Culture on Sabouraud's medium is diagnostic

- ■ Differential Diagnosis
  - Psoriasis
  - Erythema multiforme
  - Pityriasis rosea

- ■ Treatment
  - Avoid contact with infected household pets and exchange of clothing without adequate laundering
  - Microcrystalline griseofulvin orally
  - Ketoconazole for severe, recalcitrant dermatophyte infections
  - Topical antifungals in combination with steroid creams may be useful for acutely inflamed lesions

14

Tinea Cruris

- ■ Essentials of Diagnosis
  - Marked pruritus in intertriginous areas
  - Peripherally spreading, sharply demarcated, centrally clearing erythematous macular lesions with or without vesicle formation
  - May have associated tinea infection of feet
  - Examination of scraping with 10% potassium hydroxide demonstrates hyphae; culture is diagnostic

- ■ Differential Diagnosis
  - Candidiasis
  - Seborrheic dermatitis
  - Intertrigo
  - Psoriasis
  - Erythrasma
  - Tinea versicolor

- ■ Treatment
  - Application of drying powder and wearing loose-fitting underwear are important general measures
  - Oral griseofulvin may be prescribed for severe cases
  - Topical fungicides, including tolnaftate, clotrimazole, and similar agents, are highly effective

14

Tinea Manuum & Tinea Pedis (Dermatophytosis, Tinea of Palms & Soles, "Athlete's Foot")

■ Essentials of Diagnosis

- Most often presents as asymptomatic scaling
- Pruritus, burning, and stinging of interdigital webs, palms, and soles
- Deep vesicles in acute stage
- Exfoliation, fissuring, and maceration in subacute or chronic stages
- Skin scrapings examined microscopically in 10% potassium hydroxide demonstrate hyphae

■ Differential Diagnosis

- Candidiasis
- Intertrigo
- Psoriasis
- Eczema
- Scabies
- Contact dermatitis
- Gram-negative toe web infections

■ Treatment

- Personal hygiene essential factor for prevention
- Topical miconazole or clotrimazole highly effective
- Oral griseofulvin for cases resistant to topical therapy; oral ketoconazole or cases resistant to griseofulvin
- Aluminum subacetate soaks may be effective during acute phase

14

Dermatophytid (Allergy or Sensitivity to Fungi)

- **Essentials of Diagnosis**
  - A rare disorder that causes vesicles on the hand and feet
  - Pruritic, grouped vesicular lesions involving the sides and flexor aspects of the fingers and palms
  - Sensitivity reaction to a fungal infection elsewhere on the body, usually the feet
  - Trichophytin skin test positive; fungus not demonstrable in dermatophytid lesions

- **Differential Diagnosis**
  - Contact dermatitis
  - Dyshidrosis
  - Atopic dermatitis

- **Treatment**
  - Intralesional medium-potency steroids such as triamcinolone
  - Oral griseofulvin or topical antifungal medications are indicated for treating primary causative fungal infection

Tinea Unguium & Candidal Onychomycosis

- ■ Essentials of Diagnosis
  - Lusterless, brittle, hypertrophic, friable nails
  - Fungus demonstrated in nail section or nail dust by microscopy or culture

- ■ Differential Diagnosis
  - Psoriasis involving nails
  - Lichen planus
  - Trauma to nails
  - Hyperthyroidism

- ■ Treatment
  - Long-term use of full doses of griseofulvin; ketoconazole at high doses is more effective, though adrenal and liver side effects may limit usage
  - Ciclopirox, a topical fungicidal cream containing an agent to penetrate nails, may be more effective than other topical agents
  - Oral itraconazole may also be effective

Tinea Versicolor (Pityriasis Versicolor)

- **Essentials of Diagnosis**
  - A mild superficial infection due to a yeast, *Malassezia furfur (Pityrosporum orbiculare)*
  - Pale macules that will not tan; usually nonpruritic
  - Velvety, chamois-colored macules that scale with scraping
  - Tendency for truncal involvement
  - Microscopic examination of scales in 10% potassium hydroxide demonstrate large hyphae and spores of *M furfur*

- **Differential Diagnosis**
  - Vitiligo
  - Seborrheic dermatitis

- **Treatment**
  - Proper skin hygiene
  - Topical selenium sulfide suspension
  - Sulfur-salicylic acid soap or shampoo
  - Oral ketoconazole in selected cases is highly effective

Cutaneous Candidiasis (Moniliasis)

- ■ Essentials of Diagnosis
  - • Severe pruritus of vulva, anus, or intertriginous zones
  - • Superficial, denuded, beefy-red areas with or without satellite vesicles and pustules
  - • Whitish, curd-like concretions found particularly on oral and vaginal mucous membranes
  - • May be associated with underlying immunosuppression, such as HIV infection (especially oral and esophageal involvement), or with diabetes or pregnancy
  - • Microscopic examination of scales or curd in 10% potassium hydroxide demonstrates short hyphae and budding cells

- ■ Differential Diagnosis
  - • Intertrigo
  - • Seborrheic dermatitis
  - • Tinea cruris
  - • Erythrasma
  - • Psoriasis

- ■ Treatment
  - • Discontinue broad-spectrum antibiotics if thought to be contributing to fungal infection and if clinically prudent to do so; if it is not possible to discontinue antibiotics, administer oral nystatin or ketoconazole concomitantly with antibiotic
  - • Topical miconazole or clotrimazole effective in most cases
  - • Systemic oral fluconazole or ketoconazole for chronic, recurrent, or recalcitrant candidiasis, particularly vulvovaginal or esophageal involvement

14

Scabies

■ **Essentials of Diagnosis**

- Nocturnal pruritus
- Pruritic vesicles and pustules in "runs" or "galleries," especially on the sides of fingers and heels of palms
- Mites, ova, and brown dots of feces caused by infestation with *Sarcoptes scabiei* are visible microscopically
- Usually does not occur above the neck

■ **Differential Diagnosis**

- Other types of pediculosis
- Pruritus due to any other etiology

■ **Treatment**

- Treat all infested family members
- Launder or dry clean bedding and clothing
- Disinfestation with permethrin 5% applied from the neck down overnight

Pediculosis (Lice)

- ■ Essentials of Diagnosis
  - A parasitic infestation of the skin involving the scalp, trunk, or pubic areas
  - Pruritus with excoriation
  - Nits found on hair shaft; body lice identified on seams of clothing
  - Occasionally, sky-blue macules (maculae ceruleae) on the inner thighs or lower abdomen in association with pubic louse infestation

- ■ Differential Diagnosis
  - Seborrheic dermatitis
  - Scabies
  - Anogenital pruritus
  - Eczema

- ■ Treatment
  - Treat all infested family members
  - Disinfect clothing, combs, and brushes
  - Disinfestation with permethrin 5%
  - Permethrin 1% cream rinse effective for head lice and eggs
  - Fine-tooth combing of hair is essential to remove nits

14

Skin Lesions Due to Other Arthropods

- ■ Essentials of Diagnosis
    - • Arthropods that bite humans include mosquitoes, ticks, mites, biting flies, fleas, bedbugs; spiders rarely attack humans
    - • Localized rash with pruritus; reaction often delayed 1–24 hours
    - • Lesions resembling furuncles are noted and contain live arthropods
    - • Tender erythematous patches that migrate ("larva migrans")
    - • Generalized urticaria or erythema multiforme may be found
    - • Diagnosis aided by history of exposure to arthropods and by considering patient's activities and occupation

- ■ Differential Diagnosis
    - • Erythema multiforme
    - • Urticaria
    - • Pediculosis
    - • Fungal or parasitic dermatoses

- ■ Treatment
    - • Removal of living arthropods with tweezers following application of alcohol
    - • Topical steroids or crotamiton is symptomatically effective as it contains both an antipruritic and miticide
    - • Intralesional steroids for persistent lesions
    - • Papain powder is effective for stings
    - • Immunotherapy for patients at risk for anaphylaxis

14

Serum Sickness

- **Essentials of Diagnosis**
  - Fever and malaise
  - Skin rash, usually urticarial
  - Local or generalized lymphadenopathy, polyarthralgia, or polyarthritis are frequent associated findings
  - Glomerulonephritis, with red cell casts on urinalysis, may be present
  - Serum complement falls temporarily during maximal symptoms
  - History of recent treatment with a drug—frequently a penicillin or sulfonamide—is a common association

- **Differential Diagnosis**
  - Rheumatoid arthritis
  - Lupus erythematosus
  - Other systemic vasculitides
  - Hepatitis prodrome
  - Rheumatic fever

- **Treatment**
  - Discontinue offending drug
  - Systemic corticosteroids for severe symptoms

14

Keratoacanthoma

- **Essentials of Diagnosis**
  - Usually acts in a benign fashion but should be treated as if it is a skin cancer
  - Rapidly enlarging, erythematous nodule containing a central plug of keratin material
  - Most are solitary, though occasionally multiple lesions may be present
  - Associated with sun exposure with predilection for sun-exposed areas of the body
  - May regress spontaneously though usually results in scar formation
  - Histologic picture is characteristic though may be difficult to distinguish from well-differentiated squamous cell carcinomas

- **Differential Diagnosis**
  - Actinic keratosis
  - Bowen's disease
  - Basal cell carcinoma
  - Squamous cell skin cancer

- **Treatment**
  - Surgical excision important both for differentiation from other malignant processes and because it provides better cosmetic result than spontaneous regression
  - Where scar formation is unacceptable, as in face, intralesional fluorouracil may be effective

14

Actinic Keratosis (Senile or Solar Keratoses)

- Essentials of Diagnosis
  - Multiple firm, sharply defined papules with a rough, keratotic surface, frequently with an erythematous base
  - Arise in previously sun-damaged skin
  - Biopsy is diagnostic
  - In occasional patients, may transform into squamous cell carcinomas

- Differential Diagnosis
  - Squamous cell carcinoma

- Treatment
  - Most lesions may be treated satisfactorily by curettage with electrodesiccation, cautery, or cryotherapy with liquid nitrogen
  - When there is concern regarding malignant transformation, the lesions should be excised or biopsied
  - Multiple lesions may be treated with topical fluorouracil

14

Basal Cell Carcinoma (Basal Cell Epithelioma)

- ■ Essentials of Diagnosis
  - • Sun-exposed areas in fair-skinned individuals
  - • Slow-growing, translucent papule associated with telangiectasias on the surface and often central crusting or ulceration
  - • Sclerosing variant presents with yellowish, sclerotic plaque mimicking scleroderma or scar
  - • Multicentric variant presents as multiple lesions with inflammatory plaque-like appearance
  - • Basal cell nevi syndrome is characterized by autosomal dominant inheritance of multiple basal cell carcinomas with appearance beginning in childhood; lesions are widespread and not necessarily confined to sun-exposed areas
  - • May invade and destroy underlying tissues with rare metastasis

- ■ Differential Diagnosis
  - • Sclerosing variant may resemble scleroderma or scar

- ■ Treatment
  - • Smaller lesions are treated effectively with simple surgical excision, curettage, or electrodesiccation
  - • Recurrent or irregularly defined tumors may be resected by Mohs's microscopically controlled excisional surgery

14

Squamous Cell Carcinoma

- **Essentials of Diagnosis**
    - Erythematous papules enlarging to scaling nodule with ulceration
    - Increased incidence in fair-skinned individuals with predilection for sun-exposed areas of the skin
    - Often arises from preexisting, premalignant lesions, particularly actinic keratoses
    - Histologic examination is diagnostic

- **Differential Diagnosis**
    - Actinic keratosis
    - Bowen's disease
    - Basal cell carcinoma

- **Treatment**
    - Surgical excision with clear margins is essential
    - Mohs's microscopically controlled microsurgery may be necessary for complicated lesions
    - Follow-up for recurrence is essential

14

Malignant Melanoma

- **Essentials of Diagnosis**
  - Tumor of the melanocyte system with heterogeneous presentation manifested as pigmented macules, papules, or nodules occurring commonly but not exclusively in sun-exposed areas of the skin
  - Superficial spreading melanoma characterized by variation in color, ranging from black to dark brown, but also red, white, and blue
  - Thickness and surface extent of tumor determines prognosis and therapy; depth greater than 0.75 mm has worse prognosis with likelihood of metastases, but overall area correlates best with outcome
  - Histology is diagnostic

- **Differential Diagnosis**
  - Freckle or nevi
  - Ecchymosis under nail bed

- **Treatment**
  - Excision with appropriate margins based on thickness of tumor is mandatory
  - Metastatic work-up prior to excision will determine prognosis and therapy

14

Androgenetic Alopecia (Male Pattern Baldness)

- ■ Essentials of Diagnosis
  - Hair loss without scarring
  - Recession of the frontal and temporal hairline and vertex thinning are patterns found in men
  - Diffuse hair loss is manifested in women even without underlying systemic illness as described below
  - No evidence of endocrine abnormalities
  - Genetic predisposing factors
  - Endocrine abnormalities such as hypothyroidism, hyperthyroidism, iron deficiency anemia, hypopituitarism, and hypoparathyroidism should be ruled out
  - Sudden appearance of hair loss in a woman may suggest endocrine dysfunction, particularly when associated with other signs of virilization

- ■ Differential Diagnosis
  - Alopecia areata
  - Telogen effluvium
  - Scarring alopecia
  - Traction alopecia due to tight braiding or use of tight hair rollers

- ■ Treatment
  - Topical minoxidil 2% may be applied twice daily to affected areas in order to decrease hair loss as well as stimulate new hair growth, particularly over the vertex of the scalp; 50% of patients report noticeable hair growth following one year of treatment
  - Modalities such as hair transplantation and scalp reduction may provide acceptable results

14

Hirsutism

- ■ Essentials of Diagnosis
  - Increased hair growth in androgen-dependent areas only
  - Excessive androgen states associated with such conditions as polycystic ovary syndrome (Stein-Leventhal), ovarian tumors, congenital adrenal hyperplasia, hyperprolactinemia, acromegaly, and virilizing drugs must be considered
  - Free testosterone and dehydroepiandrosterone sulfate elevated in ovarian and adrenal tumors; luteinizing hormone to follicle-stimulating hormone ratio is greater than 2 in Stein-Leventhal syndrome

- ■ Differential Diagnosis
  - Hypertrichosis
  - Porphyria

- ■ Treatment
  - Treatment of underlying systemic illness if present
  - Estrogen therapy may be utilized to antagonize excessive androgen hormone
  - Shaving, waxing, electrolysis, and depilatories are effective in hair removal

14

Selected Gynecologic, Obstetric, & Breast Disorders

GYNECOLOGIC DISORDERS

Abnormal Uterine Bleeding

- **Essentials of Diagnosis**
  - Spotting at ovulation is common, but heavier or irregular bleeding warrants investigation
  - In premenopausal women, excessive bleeding may occur regularly (menorrhagia) or irregularly (dysfunctional uterine bleeding)
  - In postmenopausal women, abnormal uterine bleeding can be caused by an atrophic endometrium; endometrial proliferation, hyperplasia, cancer, or polyps; carcinoma of the cervix; and trauma
  - Anemia if bleeding is profound or chronic

- **Differential Diagnosis**
  - Ectopic pregnancy
  - Incomplete abortion
  - Pelvic neoplasm, including uterine myoma
  - Intrauterine foreign body (eg, intrauterine contraceptive device)
  - Stein-Leventhal syndrome
  - Endocrinopathies (hypothyroidism, hyperthyroidism, diabetes mellitus, pituitary disorders)
  - Use of exogenous estrogen without progestin

- **Treatment**
  - Papanicolaou smear (all ages) and endometrial biopsy (> 35 years) to exclude malignancy
  - NSAIDs can reduce blood loss in menorrhagia
  - Premenopausal: hormonal treatment (progestins limit and stabilize endometrial growth; high-dose oral contraceptives or intravenous estrogen can be used to stop active bleeding)
  - Postmenopausal: aspiration curettage frequently diagnostic and curative, followed by hormonal therapy
  - Hysterectomy for endometrial hyperplasia with atypical cells or carcinoma

Dysmenorrhea

- ■ Essentials of Diagnosis
  - Primary dysmenorrhea occurs in 50–75% of women at some time: menstrual pain associated with ovular cycles in the absence of pathologic findings; begins within 1–2 years after menarche and may increase in severity with time
  - Low, midline, wave-like, cramping pelvic pain associated with onset of menses; may radiate to the back or inner thighs and is associated with nausea, syncope, diarrhea, headache, and flushing
  - Secondary dysmenorrhea is menstrual pain for which an organic cause exists; onset may be as late as the third or fourth decade

- ■ Differential Diagnosis
  - Pelvic adhesions
  - Endometriosis
  - Uterine myoma
  - Cervical stenosis
  - Pelvic inflammatory disease
  - Intrauterine device

- ■ Treatment
  - NSAIDs should be started at the onset of bleeding and continued as needed for 2–3 days
  - Suppression of ovulation with oral contraceptives may prevent dysmenorrhea
  - In secondary dysmenorrhea, laparoscopy or hysteroscopy may be needed to determine the cause (eg, differentiate endometriosis from pelvic inflammatory disease)

15

Cervicitis

- ### Essentials of Diagnosis
  - Purulent vaginal discharge, vulvovaginal irritation, dyspareunia
  - Red, edematous cervix with purulent, often blood-streaked endocervical discharge and tenderness on cervical motion
  - Infection may follow tears during delivery or abortion or may result from a sexually transmitted pathogen such as *Neisseria gonorrhoeae, Chlamydia,* or herpesvirus
  - Infection of the cervix must be distinguished from physiologic ectopy of columnar epithelium which is common in young women

- ### Differential Diagnosis
  - Normal ovulation
  - Cervical carcinoma
  - Cervical ulcer secondary to syphilis, chancroid, or granuloma inguinale
  - Tuberculosis

- ### Treatment
  - If there is a high prevalence of sexually transmitted diseases in the population, treat empirically for *Neisseria gonorrhoeae* and *Chlamydia* with antimicrobials (eg, ciprofloxacin plus azithromycin)
  - Sexual partner should be treated
  - Electrocautery or cryosurgery for chronic cases
  - Serologic testing for concomitant subclinical syphilis and AIDS counseling

15

Vaginitis

- ■ Essentials of Diagnosis
  - Vaginal burning, pain, pruritus, or unusually profuse, malodorous discharge
  - Inflammation may result from allergic reactions to vaginal contraceptives, friction of coitus, tampons, douches, or infection
  - Common infectious causes include *Candida albicans, Trichomonas vaginalis,* bacterial vaginosis (polymicrobial infection with *Gardnerella* and other anaerobes), condylomata acuminata
  - Laboratory studies are usually diagnostic: wet preparation may reveal motile organisms with flagella (*Trichomonas vaginalis*); KOH preparation may demonstrate filaments and spores (*Candida albicans*)

- ■ Differential Diagnosis
  - Atrophic vaginitis
  - Cervicitis
  - Ovulation
  - Cervical carcinoma
  - Syphilis

- ■ Treatment
  - Culture cervix for *Neisseria gonorrhoeae* and *Chlamydia* if patient at risk for STDs
  - For *T vaginalis:* metronidazole (2 g as a single dose) for both patient and partner
  - For *C albicans:* antifungal (eg, clotrimazole) vaginal cream or suppository
  - For bacterial vaginosis: metronidazole (500 mg twice daily for 7 days)
  - For condylomata acuminata: topical application of podophyllum resin in tincture of benzoin or trichloroacetic acid; cryotherapy with liquid nitrogen

15

Myoma of the Uterus (Fibroid Tumor, Fibromyoma)

- ■ Essentials of Diagnosis
  - Irregular enlargement of uterus, often asymptomatic
  - Urinary frequency, heavy or irregular vaginal bleeding, dysmenorrhea, anemia in some patients
  - Acute and recurrent pelvic pain if the tumor becomes twisted on its pedicle or infarcted
  - Pressure symptoms on bladder or bowel
  - Benign tumor may be intramural, submucosal, subserous, intraligamentous, cervical, or parasitic (ie, deriving its blood supply from an adjacent organ)
  - Pelvic ultrasound confirms presence and monitors growth

- ■ Differential Diagnosis
  - Leiomyosarcoma of the uterus
  - Pregnancy
  - Adenomyosis
  - Ovarian adenocarcinoma
  - Endometriosis
  - Dysfunctional uterine bleeding due to other cause

- ■ Treatment
  - Papanicolaou smear and endometrial biopsy to exclude malignancy
  - Small asymptomatic myomas may be observed at regular intervals
  - For marked anemia, intramuscular progesterone or danazol will slow or stop bleeding
  - Myomectomy in patients who develop a myoma during childbearing years
  - Hysterectomy for refractory pain, rapid or large growth, severe bleeding, or symptoms of pressure on bladder and bowel

15

Endometriosis

- ### Essentials of Diagnosis
  - Aberrant growth of endometrium outside the uterus, particularly in the ovaries and dependent parts of the pelvis
  - Constant aching pain, beginning 2–7 days before the onset of menses and becoming increasingly severe until flow decreases
  - Pelvic examination may reveal indurated nodules in the cul-de-sac, especially if the examination is done at the onset of menstruation
  - Bowel invasion by endometrial tissue may produce blood in the stool that must be distinguished from bowel neoplasm
  - Ultrasound examination will often reveal complex fluid-filled masses that cannot be distinguished from neoplasms
  - Laparoscopy confirms the diagnosis

- ### Differential Diagnosis
  - Pelvic inflammatory disease
  - Ovarian neoplasms
  - Uterine myomas

- ### Treatment
  - NSAIDs
  - Oral contraceptives or medroxyprogesterone for 6–9 months
  - GnRH analogues (eg, nafarelin nasal spray or leuprolide) to suppress ovulation
  - In patients under age 35, surgical resection of lesions with bipolar coagulation or laser vaporization at laparoscopy
  - In patients over 35 with disabling pain, consider bilateral salpingo-oophorectomy and hysterectomy followed by estrogen replacement therapy

15

Pelvic Inflammatory Disease
(PID, Salpingitis, Endometritis)

- ■ Essentials of Diagnosis
  - Polymicrobial infection of the upper genital tract associated with *Neisseria gonorrhoeae* and *Chlamydia trachomatis* as well as endogenous organisms, including anaerobes, *Haemophilus influenzae,* enteric gram-negative rods, and streptococci
  - Most common in young, nulliparous, sexually active women with multiple partners
  - Lower abdominal or pelvic pain, fever, chills; adnexal and cervical motion tenderness
  - Cervical or vaginal discharge; leukocytosis and elevated sedimentation rate
  - Right upper quadrant pain (Fitzhugh-Curtis syndrome) may result from associated perihepatitis
  - Laparoscopy reveals findings consistent with pelvic inflammatory disease; pelvic ultrasound may demonstrate a tubo-ovarian abscess

- ■ Differential Diagnosis
  - Appendicitis
  - Acute enteritis
  - Ruptured ovarian cyst or tumor
  - Ovarian torsion
  - Septic abortion
  - Ectopic pregnancy
  - Endometriosis
  - Degeneration of uterine myoma
  - Tuberculous salpingitis

15

- ■ Treatment
  - Oral antibiotics covering *N gonorrhoeae* and *Chlamydia* for mildly ill patients; sexual partner should be treated
  - Hospitalization and intravenous antibiotics for toxic or pregnant patients
  - Surgical or percutaneous drainage of tubo-ovarian abscess if present
  - Screening serologic testing for syphilis and AIDS counseling
  - Use of barrier contraceptive methods may provide significant protection against PID

Genital & Uterine Prolapse

- **Essentials of Diagnosis**
  - Cystocele, rectocele, and enterocele are vaginal hernias commonly seen in multiparous women
  - Cystocele is a hernia of the bladder wall into the vagina; it may be accompanied by a urethrocele (a sagging of the urethra following its detachment from the pubic symphysis during childbirth)
  - Rectocele is a herniation of the terminal rectum into the posterior vagina
  - Enterocele is a hernia containing small intestine and protruding into the posterior vaginal vault
  - Uterine prolapse may be slight (uterus descends only part way down the vagina), moderate (uterus descends to the introitus and cervix extends beyond), or marked (the entire cervix and uterus protrude beyond the introitus and the vagina is inverted
  - Uterine prolapse most commonly occurs as a delayed result of childbirth injury to the pelvic floor; attenuation of the pelvic structures with aging can accelerate the development of prolapse

- **Differential Diagnosis**
  - Vaginal or cervical neoplasm
  - Rectal carcinoma

- **Treatment**
  - Supportive measures including a high-fiber diet, weight reduction in obese patients, and limitation of straining and lifting
  - Pessaries may reduce cystocele, rectocele, or enterocele
  - Corrective surgery for significant cystocele, rectocele, or enterocele
  - Consider vaginal pessary or hysterectomy for uterine prolapse

15

Spontaneous Abortion

- **Essentials of Diagnosis**
  - Vaginal bleeding with low abdominal or pelvic pain and cramping before the 20th week of pregnancy; disappearance of signs and symptoms of pregnancy
  - Threatened abortion: bleeding or cramping occurs, but pregnancy continues
  - Inevitable abortion: cervix is dilated and membranes rupture, but products of conception have not passed
  - Incomplete abortion: some portion of the products of conception are expelled but others (eg, placenta) remain in the uterus
  - Complete abortion: fetus and placenta are completely expelled
  - Serum β-hCG low or falling
  - Pelvic ultrasonography confirms presence or loss of gestational sac

- **Differential Diagnosis**
  - Incompetent cervix
  - Ectopic pregnancy
  - Menorrhagia
  - Gestational trophoblastic neoplasia
  - Pedunculated uterine myoma
  - Cervical neoplasm

- **Treatment**
  - For threatened abortion, bed rest for 24–48 hours followed by gradual resumption of usual activities; for patients with incompetent cervix, cerclage and restriction of all activities
  - For inevitable or incomplete abortion, D&C with removal of products of conception (send tissue for pathologic examination)
  - After complete abortion, administer Rh_o immune globulin to Rh-negative mothers and document decreasing serum β-hCG levels

15

Menopausal Syndrome

- ■ Essentials of Diagnosis
  - Cessation of menses due to aging or to bilateral oophorectomy
  - Menstrual irregularity; hot flushes and night sweats in 80% of women; dyspareunia
  - Decreased vaginal lubrication; thinned vaginal mucosa; dyspareunia
  - Elevation of serum FSH and LH levels

- ■ Differential Diagnosis
  - Hyperthyroidism or hypothyroidism
  - Uterine neoplasm
  - Sjögren's syndrome
  - Carcinoid syndrome

- ■ Treatment
  - Short-term estrogen therapy with or without progestins for relief of menopausal symptoms
  - Long-acting progestins if estrogens cannot be tolerated
  - Consider long-term estrogen or progesterone replacement therapy to decrease risk of myocardial infarction, improve lipids, and prevent osteoporosis
  - Careful follow-up of breast and uterine examination for development of previously subclinical malignancy

15

OBSTETRIC DISORDERS

Ectopic Pregnancy

- **Essentials of Diagnosis**
  - Implantation of the ovum outside the cavity of the uterus (ie, uterine tube, peritoneum, abdominal viscera, ovary, or cervix)
  - Amenorrhea, irregular vaginal bleeding, severe pelvic pain, symptoms of pregnancy
  - Tenderness on pelvic examination; mass sometimes palpable outside uterus
  - Shock if ectopic pregnancy ruptures
  - Serum β-hCG lower than expected for normal pregnancy, or failure to rise appropriately
  - Pelvic ultrasound should demonstrate a gestational sac by 6 weeks following the last menstrual period, so an empty uterine cavity at 6–7 weeks is highly suggestive
  - Transvaginal ultrasound may demonstrate an extrauterine pregnancy; laparoscopy confirms presence of ectopic pregnancy and allows surgical removal

- **Differential Diagnosis**
  - Intrauterine pregnancy
  - Appendicitis
  - Pelvic inflammatory disease
  - Gestational trophoblastic neoplasia
  - Ruptured corpus luteum cyst
  - Urinary calculi

- **Treatment**
  - Methotrexate for unruptured pregnancies less than 3.5 cm with no active bleeding
  - Surgical removal of larger or complicated ectopic pregnancies
  - Administer Rh_o immune globulin to Rh-negative patients
  - Careful observation and early ultrasound confirmation of future pregnancies (repeat tubal pregnancy occurs in about 12% of cases)

15

Pregnancy-Induced Hypertension (Preeclampsia-Eclampsia)

- **Essentials of Diagnosis**
  - Preeclampsia is the triad of hypertension, proteinuria, and edema during pregnancy; eclampsia is the addition of seizures to this triad
  - Affects 7% of pregnant women; may occur any time between 20 weeks of gestation and 6 weeks postpartum
  - Associated signs and symptoms include headache, blurred vision, abdominal pain, altered mentation, hyperreflexia; laboratory findings include thrombocytopenia, hyperuricemia
  - Increased incidence in primiparas and patients with hypertension, diabetes, chronic renal disease, and in patients with autoimmune disorders

- **Differential Diagnosis**
  - Chronic hypertension
  - Chronic renal disease
  - Primary seizure disorders
  - Hemolytic uremic syndrome

- **Treatment**
  - Early recognition, salt restriction, bed rest, and close monitoring of blood pressure and proteinuria in mild cases
  - Hospitalization for women with moderate or severe preeclampsia or those with unreliable home situations
  - Antihypertensive therapy
  - For eclampsia, a medical emergency, intravenous magnesium sulfate and diazepam
  - Only cure is termination of pregnancy as soon as it is possible for the fetus to survive

15

BREAST DISORDERS

Mammary Dysplasia (Fibrocystic Breast Disease)

- ■ Essentials of Diagnosis
  - Painful, often multiple, usually bilateral masses in breast
  - Rapid fluctuation in size of masses
  - Pain or increase in size during premenstrual phase of cycle
  - Common age 30–50; rare in postmenopausal women

- ■ Differential Diagnosis
  - Breast carcinoma
  - Benign tumor of the breast

- ■ Treatment
  - Mammography, biopsy of suspicious lesions to exclude carcinoma
  - Regular breast self-examination with attention to any new mass
  - Supportive brassiere (night and day)
  - Danazol (100–200 mg twice daily) for severe pain
  - Vitamin E supplementation and discontinuation of caffeine may be helpful

Puerperal Mastitis

- ■ Essentials of Diagnosis
  - Occurs in nursing mothers within 3 months after delivery
  - Unilateral inflammation of the breast
  - Sore or fissured nipple with surrounding redness, tenderness, induration, warmth, fever
  - Increased incidence in first-time mothers
  - *Staphylococcus aureus* is usual causative agent
  - May progress to breast abscess if untreated within first 24 hours

- ■ Differential Diagnosis
  - Local irritation or trauma
  - Benign or malignant tumors
  - Subareolar abscess (occurs in nonlactating women)
  - Fat necrosis

- ■ Treatment
  - Dicloxacillin or first-generation cephalosporin
  - Regular emptying of the breast by nursing
  - Expression of any remaining milk either by hand or with a mechanical suction device
  - Incision and drainage of abscesses

Gynecomastia

- **Essentials of Diagnosis**
  - Glandular enlargement of the male breast
  - Often asymmetric or unilateral and may be tender
  - Nipple discharge may be present
  - Common in puberty and among elderly men
  - Multiple causes include obesity, androgen resistance, hyperprolactinemia, hyperthyroidism, hypogonadism, chronic liver disease, adrenal tumors, testicular tumors, bronchogenic carcinoma, elaborating ectopic gonadotropins and drugs (eg, alcohol, amiodarone, diazepam, digoxin, isoniazid, ketoconazole, marijuana, omeprazole, tricyclic antidepressants)

- **Differential Diagnosis**
  - Associations noted above
  - Benign or malignant tumors of the breast

- **Treatment**
  - Careful testicular examination; chest x-ray to rule out bronchogenic carcinoma; measurement of β-hCG, LH, testosterone, and estradiol may be indicated to rule out underlying disorder
  - Needle biopsy of suspicious areas of breast enlargement
  - Remove offending drug or treat underlying condition; reassurance if idiopathic
  - Consider surgical correction for severe cases

15

16

Common Surgical Disorders

Abdominal Aortic Aneurysm

- **Essentials of Diagnosis**
  - Most are asymptomatic and detected incidentally at physical examination or sonography
  - Pulsating upper abdominal mass, mild midabdominal or lower back discomfort in 25–33% of cases
  - More than 90% originate below the renal arteries
  - Back or abdominal pain often precedes rupture
  - 90% leak into left retroperitoneum; 10% rupture anteriorly, causing sudden death

- **Differential Diagnosis**
  - Gastrointestinal malignancy
  - Pancreatic pseudocyst
  - Multiple myeloma
  - Musculoskeletal causes of back pain

- **Treatment**
  - In asymptomatic patients, depending on age and presence of other medical conditions, surgery is recommended when the aneurysm is 5 or 6 cm
  - Surgical resection may even be beneficial for aneurysms as small as 4 cm
  - In symptomatic patients, urgent repair is recommended irrespective of size
  - For rupture, emergent surgical repair
  - Endovascular repair if anatomy of aneurysm is suitable

Pharyngoesophageal Diverticulum (Zenker's Diverticulum)

- **Essentials of Diagnosis**
  - Dysphagia worsening as more is eaten; regurgitation of undigested food, halitosis
  - Gurgling sounds in the neck on auscultation
  - Barium swallow confirms diagnosis

- **Differential Diagnosis**
  - Esophageal, mediastinal, or neck tumor
  - Cricopharyngeal achalasia (occasionally associated)
  - Esophageal web
  - Achalasia or lower esophageal stricture

- **Treatment**
  - Surgical excision with cricopharyngeal myotomy

Obstruction of the Small Intestine

- ■ Essentials of Diagnosis
  - Crampy abdominal pain, vomiting, abdominal distention, constipation or obstipation
  - Distended, tender abdomen with or without peritoneal signs; high-pitched tinkling or peristaltic rushes audible
  - Adhesions, hernias the commonest causes
  - Dilated small bowel on x-ray, with air-fluid levels

- ■ Differential Diagnosis
  - Adynamic ileus due to any cause (eg, hypokalemia, pancreatitis, nephrolithiasis)
  - Colonic obstruction
  - Intestinal pseudo-obstruction

- ■ Treatment
  - Nasogastric suction
  - Fluid and electrolyte (especially potassium) replacement
  - Surgical exploration for suspected strangulation, or obstruction not responsive to conservative therapy

16

Functional Obstruction
(Adynamic Ileus, Paralytic Ileus)

- **Essentials of Diagnosis**
  - Continuous abdominal pain, distention, vomiting, and obstipation
  - History of precipitating factor (recent surgery, peritonitis, other serious medical illness, anticholinergic drugs, hypokalemia)
  - Minimal abdominal tenderness; decreased to absent bowel sounds
  - Radiographic evidence of gas and fluid in small and large intestine

- **Differential Diagnosis**
  - Mechanical obstruction due to any cause
  - Specific diseases associated with functional obstruction, ie, perforated viscus, pancreatitis, cholecystitis, appendicitis, nephrolithiasis
  - Colonic pseudo-obstruction

- **Treatment**
  - Restriction of oral intake; nasogastric suction in severe cases
  - Attention to electrolyte and fluid imbalance (ie, hypokalemia, dehydration)

16

Acute Appendicitis

- ■ **Essentials of Diagnosis**
  - Should be suspected in all patients with unexplained abdominal pain
  - Abdominal pain, initially poorly localized or periumbilical, then migrating to right lower quadrant
  - Anorexia, nausea, vomiting, constipation typical, but many variations
  - Right lower quadrant tenderness (McBurney's point) with or without peritoneal signs, eg, localized rigidity; low-grade fever
  - Leukocytosis; microscopic hematuria or pyuria common
  - Sonographic visualization of appendix confirmatory but unnecessary

- ■ **Differential Diagnosis**
  - Gastroenteritis
  - Pelvic disease in women (ie, ectopic pregnancy, pelvic inflammatory disease, ovarian cyst)
  - Nephrolithiasis
  - Pyelonephritis
  - Crohn's disease
  - Meckel's diverticulitis
  - Mesenteric adenitis
  - Acute cholecystitis
  - Right lower lobe pneumonia

- ■ **Treatment**
  - Appendectomy

16

Mesenteric Lymphadenitis

- ■ Essentials of Diagnosis
  - Acute abdominal or periumbilical pain; anorexia, nausea, vomiting, high fever may be seen
  - Right lower quadrant tenderness with little peritoneal irritation
  - Leukocytosis
  - History of recent or concurrent upper respiratory or diarrheal illness common
  - Usually a self-limiting illness caused by viruses, bacteria, parasites, toxins, or unknown agents

- ■ Differential Diagnosis
  - Appendicitis
  - Meckel's diverticulitis
  - Nephrolithiasis
  - Right lower lobe pneumonia

- ■ Treatment
  - Observation with supportive care
  - Surgical exploration if appendicitis cannot be excluded
  - Treat underlying infection if disease is not self-limited and if causative organism is known

Diverticulitis

- ■ Essentials of Diagnosis
  - Most diverticula are asymptomatic (diverticulosis), though hemorrhage may occur from those on the right colon
  - Acute, intermittent, cramping left lower abdominal pain; constipation or alternating constipation and diarrhea
  - Fever, tenderness in left lower quadrant, with palpable abdominal mass in some patients
  - Leukocytosis
  - Radiographic evidence of diverticula, thickened interhaustral folds, narrowed lumen

- ■ Differential Diagnosis
  - Colorectal carcinoma
  - Appendicitis
  - Strangulating colonic obstruction
  - Colitis due to any cause
  - Pelvic inflammatory disease
  - Ruptured ectopic pregnancy or ovarian cyst

- ■ Treatment
  - High-residue diet, stool softener, psyllium mucilloid for chronic therapy
  - Metronidazole plus either ciprofloxacin or trimethoprim-sulfamethoxazole for mild symptoms
  - Nasogastric suction and broad-spectrum, intravenous antibiotics for patients requiring hospitalization
  - Percutaneous catheter drainage for abdominal abscess
  - Laparotomy for refractory cases, obstruction, fistula, perforation

16

Pancreatic Pseudocyst

- ■ Essentials of Diagnosis
    - Collection of pancreatic fluid in or around the pancreas; may occur as a complication of acute or chronic pancreatitis
    - Characterized by epigastric pain, tenderness, fever, and occasionally a palpable mass
    - Leukocytosis, persistent serum amylase elevation
    - Pancreatic cyst demonstrated by CT scan
    - Complications include hemorrhage, infection, rupture, fistula formation, and obstruction of surrounding organs

- ■ Differential Diagnosis
    - Pancreatic phlegmon or abscess
    - Resolving pancreatitis
    - Pancreatic carcinoma

- ■ Treatment
    - Up to two-thirds may spontaneously resolve
    - Percutaneous catheter drainage with avoidance of food and parenteral nutritional support effective in many cases
    - Decompression into an adjacent hollow viscus (cystojejunostomy or cystogastrostomy) may be necessary
    - Octreotide to inhibit pancreatic secretion; avoidance of alcohol

Inguinal Hernia

- ## Essentials of Diagnosis
  - Lump or swelling in the groin, sometimes associated with sudden pain and bulging during heavy lifting or straining
  - An indirect inguinal hernia (most common) occurs when abdominal contents enter the previously empty peritoneal diverticulum through dilation of the internal inguinal ring
  - A direct inguinal hernia results from protrusion of the abdominal contents through a weakening of the transversalis fascia in Hesselbach's area
  - A femoral hernia is an acquired protrusion of a peritoneal sac through the femoral ring
  - Contents of a reducible hernia return to the abdomen spontaneously or with manual pressure; an irreducible (incarcerated) hernia cannot be returned to the abdomen
  - In a strangulated hernia, blood supply to the hernia sac has been compromised and gangrene has occurred

- ## Differential Diagnosis
  - Hydrocele
  - Varicocele
  - Lymphadenopathy or abscess of the groin
  - Lipoma of the spermatic cord
  - Hematoma following trauma
  - Intestinal obstruction of other cause

- ## Treatment
  - Elective surgical repair for reducible hernias
  - Emergent repair for incarcerated or strangulated hernias

16

Intestinal Ischemia

- **Essentials of Diagnosis**
  - Acute intestinal ischemia may result from (1) embolic occlusion of the visceral branches of the abdominal aorta (eg, in patients with mitral valvular disease, atrial fibrillation, or left ventricular thrombus); (2) thrombosis of one or more of the visceral vessels (ie, in patients with atherosclerotic occlusive changes); or (3) nonocclusive mesenteric vascular insufficiency (eg, in patients with congestive heart failure or hypovolemic shock)
  - Acute onset of severe, diffuse abdominal pain associated with intestinal bleeding, high leukocyte count, and minimal or no findings on abdominal examination
  - Lactic acidosis, hypotension, and abdominal distention are late findings suggesting bowel infarction rather than ischemia
  - Chronic intestinal ischemia results from atherosclerotic occlusive lesions at or close to the origins of the superior mesenteric, celiac, and inferior mesenteric arteries, leading to a significant reduction of blood flow to the intestines.
  - Epigastric or periumbilical postprandial pains that last for 1–3 hours; patients limit oral intake to avoid pain resulting in significant weight loss in such patients
  - Ischemic colitis develops when the diminished circulation is most prominent in the distribution of the inferior mesenteric artery; patients may have episodic bouts of crampy lower abdominal pain associated with mild, often bloody diarrhea

- **Differential Diagnosis**
  - Diverticulitis
  - Aortoenteric fistula
  - Appendicitis
  - Inflammatory bowel disease
  - Gastrointestinal malignancy
  - Vasculitis

- **Treatment**
  - Broad-spectrum antibiotics covering intestinal flora
  - Laparotomy with removal of necrotic bowel; reconstruction of superior mesenteric artery in selected patients with chronic ischemia
  - Pre- and postoperative intra-arterial infusion of papaverine if occlusion is embolic

16

Acute Cholecystitis

- **Essentials of Diagnosis**
  - Acute, steady right-sided or midabdominal pain; nausea, fatty food intolerance
  - Jaundice, fever, right upper quadrant tenderness, occasionally local rigidity, and inhibition of inspiration on deep palpation under the right subcostal margin (Murphy's sign)
  - Leukocytosis, slight elevation in liver function studies and amylase
  - Palpable gallbladder in some patients
  - Nonopacified gallbladder on radionuclide excretion scan (HIDA)
  - Gallstones on ultrasound scan

- **Differential Diagnosis**
  - Acute pancreatitis
  - Peptic ulcer disease
  - Acute appendicitis
  - Acute hepatitis
  - Right lower lobe pneumonia
  - Myocardial infarction
  - Radicular pain in thoracic dermatome

- **Treatment**
  - Withhold oral feedings, intravenous fluids, and analgesics; give parenteral antibiotics to cover coliform organisms
  - If the diagnosis of cholecystitis is made within 24–48 hours after the onset of symptoms, early cholecystectomy leads to reduced morbidity and mortality
  - If the diagnosis is delayed beyond 48 hours, surgery may be postponed for several weeks until the acute inflammation has subsided
  - Immediate cholecystectomy should be performed for evidence of perforation or gangrene; percutaneously placed cholecystostomy catheters can be used to temporize in severely ill or elderly patients with high surgical risk
  - ERCP with sphincterotomy should be performed when there is associated pancreatitis or cholangitis

16

17

Common Pediatric Disorders*

Pyloric Stenosis

- **Essentials of Diagnosis**
  - Increase in size of the muscle of the pylorus due to unknown cause; occurs in one out of 500 births, with males affected three or four times more commonly than females
  - Vomiting usually begins between 2 and 4 weeks of age and may become projectile; vomitus is rarely bilious
  - Infant is hungry and nurses avidly, but weight gain is poor and failure to thrive occurs
  - Constipation, dehydration, and hypochloremic alkalosis with hypokalemia are commonly seen
  - Palpable olive-sized mass in the subhepatic region after the child has vomited
  - "String sign" and retained gastric contents on upper gastrointestinal series; ultrasound shows a hypoechoic mass

- **Differential Diagnosis**
  - Esophageal stenosis or achalasia
  - Small bowel obstruction due to other causes
  - Adrenal insufficiency
  - Pylorospasm
  - Other causes of failure to thrive

- **Treatment**
  - Pyloromyotomy is the treatment of choice
  - Dehydration and electrolyte abnormalities should be corrected prior to surgery
  - Excellent prognosis after surgery

---

*The following common childhood diseases are discussed in other chapters: aspiration of foreign body and cystic fibrosis, Chapter 2; pharyngitis, mumps, poliomyelitis, varicella and zoster, mononucleosis, rabies, and rubella, Chapter 8; appendicitis, Chapter 16; otitis media and otitis externa, Chapter 19.

Reye's Syndrome (Encephalopathy With Fatty Degeneration of the Viscera)

■ Essentials of Diagnosis
  • Seen in patients with an upper respiratory tract infection, influenza, or chickenpox who are given salicylates
  • Vomiting, irrational behavior, progressive stupor, and coma
  • Hyperpnea, irregular respirations, dilated and sluggish pupils, evidence of cerebral edema
  • Elevated AST, ALT, and LDH, prolonged prothrombin time, normal to slightly elevated bilirubin, and variable hypoglycemia; cerebrospinal fluid usually acellular
  • Histopathology of the brain, liver, and kidney all show changes characteristic of this syndrome (microvesicular steatosis)

■ Differential Diagnosis
  • Acute toxic encephalopathy
  • Fulminant viral hepatitis
  • Meningoencephalitis due to various causes
  • Fatty acid oxidation defects

■ Treatment
  • Treatment is primarily supportive; patients should be admitted to the ICU
  • Mechanical ventilation and intracranial pressure monitoring may be needed
  • At least 70% of patients survive

Down's Syndrome

- **■ Essentials of Diagnosis**
  - Occurs in 1:600 newborns, with a higher incidence in children of mothers over 35 years of age
  - Ninety-five percent of patients have 47 chromosomes with trisomy of chromosome 21
  - Characteristic findings are small brachycephalic head, flat nasal bridge, ruddy cheeks, dry lips, short fleshy neck, epicanthic folds, and simian creases
  - One-third have congenital heart disease; leukemia is 20 times more common, and there is an increased susceptibility to infections

- **■ Differential Diagnosis**
  - The chromosome abnormalities are pathognomonic

- **■ Treatment**
  - No convincing evidence of the merit of any of the forms of general therapy that have been tried (eg, megadoses of vitamins, exercise programs)
  - Therapy is directed toward specific problems (eg, cardiac surgery, antibiotics)
  - Goal of therapy is to help affected patients develop full potential

Respiratory Syncytial Virus (RSV) Disease

- **Essentials of Diagnosis**
  - The most important cause of lower respiratory tract illness in young children, causing over 90% of cases of bronchiolitis and many cases of pneumonia
  - Epidemics in late fall to early spring; attack rates are high
  - The classic disease—bronchiolitis—is characterized by diffuse wheezing, difficulty feeding, variable fever, cough, tachypnea, hyperinflation, and retractions
  - Apnea may be the presenting symptom, especially in premature infants
  - Chest x-ray shows hyperinflation and peribronchiolar thickening
  - RSV antigen can be detected in nasal or pulmonary secretions in most patients

- **Differential Diagnosis**
  - Bronchiolitis due to other viruses or bacteria
  - Asthma
  - Foreign body aspiration
  - Chlamydial pneumonitis
  - Cystic fibrosis
  - Pertussis

- **Treatment**
  - Severely ill children should be hospitalized, given humidified oxygen, and kept in respiratory isolation
  - A trial of bronchodilator therapy is usually instituted
  - Ribavirin, given by continuous aerosolization, may be given to selected patients

17

Roseola Infantum (Exanthema Subitum)

- ### Essentials of Diagnosis
  - A benign illness caused by human herpesvirus 6 occurring primarily in children 6 months to 4 years of age (90% of cases occurring before the second year)
  - Abrupt onset of fever (as high as 40 °C) lasting up to 8 days in an otherwise mildly ill child; dissociation between systemic symptoms and febrile course
  - Fever ceases abruptly, and a characteristic rash develops in 20% of patients; rash consists of rose-pink macules or maculopapules beginning on the trunk and spreading outward with disappearance in 1–2 days
  - Absence of cough, conjunctivitis, coryza, and pharyngeal exudate
  - Rash may occur without fever

- ### Differential Diagnosis
  - Serious bacterial infections
  - Drug allergy
  - Measles
  - Rubella
  - Enterovirus infection
  - Scarlet fever
  - Toxic shock syndrome
  - Kawasaki disease

- ### Treatment
  - Supportive care only, with acetaminophen and sponge baths for the fever
  - Reassurance for the parents
  - Febrile seizures can occur, but no more commonly than with other self-limited infections

Acute Lymphoblastic Leukemia (ALL)

- **Essentials of Diagnosis**
  - ALL is the most common malignancy of childhood; peak age at onset is 4 years
  - Due to an unknown cause and results from uncontrolled proliferation of immature lymphocytes
  - Intermittent fever, bone pain, petechiae, purpura, pallor, hepatosplenomegaly, and lymphadenopathy
  - Single or multiple cytopenias are common: neutropenia, thrombocytopenia, or anemia, although very elevated lymphocyte counts may be encountered; serum uric acid and LDH often elevated
  - Diagnosis established by bone marrow examination—homogenous infiltration of more than 25% of leukemic blasts; most patients have blasts that express common ALL antigen (CALLA)

- **Differential Diagnosis**
  - EBV infection
  - CMV disease
  - Immune thrombocytopenic purpura
  - Autoimmune hemolytic anemia
  - Aplastic anemia
  - Juvenile rheumatoid arthritis
  - Pertussis, when total white blood count markedly elevated

- **Treatment**
  - Induction therapy (first month of therapy) with various agents including prednisone, vincristine, asparaginase, daunorubicin, or methotrexate
  - Consolidation phase: intrathecal chemotherapy and sometimes cranial irradiation to treat lymphoblasts that may be present in the meninges
  - Maintenance therapy with mercaptopurine, weekly methotrexate, and monthly vincristine or prednisone
  - Bone marrow transplant in selected patients
  - Children with white counts under 50,000/μL at diagnosis or those between 2 and 9 years of age have better prognoses
  - Over 70% of treated patients are cured

17

Neuroblastoma

■ **Essentials of Diagnosis**

- A tumor arising from neural crest tissue of the sympathetic ganglia or adrenal medulla; the most common solid neoplasm outside the central nervous system in children
- Fifty percent of patients diagnosed before age 2 and 90% before age 5
- Constitutional symptoms (fever, weight loss, irritability); bone pain, abdominal pain
- Adenopathy, skull masses, subcutaneous nodules, hepatomegaly, evidence of spinal cord compression
- Anemia, elevated LDH, ferritin, and urinary catecholamines; specific tumor markers include neuron-specific enolase and serum ganglioside

■ **Differential Diagnosis**

Other "small, round, blue cell" malignancies of childhood:
- Ewing's sarcoma
- Rhabdomyosarcoma
- Peripheral neuroepithelioma
- Lymphoma

■ **Treatment**

- Therapy is multimodal and involves surgery, radiation, and chemotherapy
- Prognosis depends upon age at diagnosis and stage of disease
- The overall survival in advanced disease has changed little over 20 years and remains quite low

Wilms' Tumor (Nephroblastoma)

- ■ Essentials of Diagnosis
  - This tumor, arising from the kidney, represents 6% of cancers in patients under 15 years of age; mean age at diagnosis is 3 years
  - Can occur sporadically or as part of a malformation syndrome, or cytogenic abnormality
  - Asymptomatic abdominal mass or swelling (80%), fever (25%), and hematuria (20%)
  - Hypertension, genitourinary abnormalities, aniridia, hemihypertrophy occasionally seen
  - Abdominal ultrasound or CT reveals an intrarenal mass; 10% of patients will have metastatic disease (lung or liver) at time of diagnosis

- ■ Differential Diagnosis
  - Neuroblastoma originating from the adrenal
  - Other abdominal tumors

- ■ Treatment
  - Once the diagnosis is made, almost all patients undergo surgical exploration of the abdomen with attempted excision of the tumor
  - Vincristine and dactinomycin are routinely used in all patients; doxorubicin is also administered in those with advanced disease
  - Flank irradiation is also effective in some patients

Osteosarcoma

- **Essentials of Diagnosis**
  - The sixth most common cancer in childhood but the third most common in adolescents and young adults
  - Peak occurrence during the adolescent growth spurt; males affected more commonly
  - Long tubular bones are primarily involved; in descending order of frequency: distal femur, proximal tibia, proximal humerus, and mid and proximal femur
  - Clinical manifestations include pain at the site of involvement (often following mild trauma), mass lesion, and pathologic fracture
  - Radiographs may show destruction of the bone, periosteal new bone formation, and a soft tissue mass with radial calcification
  - CT scan or MRI useful to define extent of the primary lesion; bone scan useful for detecting "skip" lesions; CT of chest essential to assess pulmonary metastases

- **Differential Diagnosis**
  - Ewing's sarcoma
  - Rhabdomyosarcoma
  - Juvenile rheumatoid arthritis
  - Osgood-Schlatter disease
  - Benign bone tumors

- **Treatment**
  - Surgical resection of the primary tumor (amputation or limb salvage)
  - Adjuvant or neoadjuvant chemotherapy with multiple agents is effective
  - Pulmonary metastases are seen in 20% at the time of diagnosis and imply a poor prognosis

17

Juvenile Rheumatoid Arthritis (Still's Disease)

- ■ Essentials of Diagnosis
  - Four patterns of disease, each with characteristic clinical manifestations:
    1. Acute febrile form characterized by an evanescent salmon-pink macular rash, oligoarticular arthritis, hepatosplenomegaly, leukocytosis, and polyserositis
    2. Polyarticular pattern resembles the adult disease, with symmetric polyarthritis, low-grade fever, fatigue, and anemia
    3. Pauciarticular pattern characterized by chronic arthritis of a few joints in asymmetric distribution; extra-articular features uncommon except for iridocyclitis (seen in 30%)
    4. Fourth pattern occurs in late childhood, affecting mainly boys; begins as a pauciarticular arthritis involving lower limbs and then progresses to involve the sacroiliac joints, lumbar and thoracic spine
  - Rheumatoid factor positive in only 15%, in whom adult rheumatoid arthritis is probably present; diagnosis based on characteristic clinical pattern

- ■ Differential Diagnosis
  - Rheumatic fever
  - Bacterial arthritis
  - Reactive arthritis due to various causes
  - Lyme disease
  - SLE
  - Dermatomyositis
  - Bone tumors

- ■ Treatment
  - Goals of treatment are to restore function, relieve pain, and maintain joint function
  - NSAIDs and physical therapy are the mainstays of treatment
  - Methotrexate, gold salts, and local corticosteroid injections are indicated for those who are still symptomatic

17

Colic

- ■ Essentials of Diagnosis
  - A "syndrome" characterized by severe and paroxysmal crying that occurs mainly in the late afternoon
  - Abdomen is distended, the facies is "pained," the fists are clenched, and the infant is unresponsive to soothing
  - Thought to be due to a disturbance in the gastrointestinal tract, but this has never been proved
  - Begins in the first few weeks of life and peaks at 2–3 months; may last into the fifth month of life
  - Diagnosis is based on the "rule of threes": a healthy infant that cries for more than 3 hours a day, for more than 3 days a week, and for more than 3 weeks

- ■ Differential Diagnosis
  - Normal crying in an infant
  - Any illness in the infant

- ■ Treatment
  - Reassurance to the parents that the infant is not "sick"
  - Education of the parents regarding the baby's cues
  - Phenobarbital elixir and dicyclomine are no longer recommended
  - Elimination of cow's milk from the formula—or from the mother's diet if she is nursing—may be indicated in refractory cases

17

Tetralogy of Fallot

- **Essentials of Diagnosis**
  - The most common type of cyanotic heart disease, accounting for 15% of all cases of congenital heart disease
  - Characterized by a ventricular septal defect, obstruction to right ventricular outflow, right ventricular hypertrophy, and overriding aorta
  - Cyanosis after the neonatal period, dyspnea on exertion, easy fatigability, growth retardation, alteration in consciousness
  - Right ventricular lift, systolic ejection murmur (rough) maximal at the left sternal border, single S_2
  - Elevated hematocrit, boot-shaped heart on chest x-ray
  - Echocardiography, cardiac catheterization, and angiocardiography all useful in confirming the diagnosis

- **Differential Diagnosis**

  Other cyanotic heart diseases:
  - Pulmonary atresia with intact ventricular septum
  - Tricuspid atresia
  - Hypoplastic left heart syndrome
  - Complete transposition of the great arteries
  - Total anomalous pulmonary venous return
  - Persistent truncus arteriosus

- **Treatment**
  - Acute treatment of cyanotic episodes includes supplemental oxygen, placing the patient in the knee-chest position, consideration of parenteral morphine sulfate and propranolol
  - Palliation (oral beta-blockers or surgical anastomosis between a systemic artery and pulmonary artery) is recommended for very small infants with severe symptoms and in those who are not candidates for complete correction
  - Total surgical correction is the treatment of choice in selected patients; these patients are still at risk for sudden death because of arrhythmias

17

Kawasaki Disease
(Mucocutaneous Lymph Node Syndrome)

- **■ Essentials of Diagnosis**
  - Illness of unknown cause characterized by prolonged fever unresponsive to antibiotics, conjunctivitis, inflamed mucous membranes, cervical lymphadenopathy, rash over the trunk and extremities, edema, and arthritis
  - Cardiovascular complications include myocarditis, pericarditis, and arteritis that predisposes to coronary artery aneurysm formation
  - Acute myocardial infarction may occur; 1–2% of patients die from this during the initial phase of the disease
  - Thrombocytosis, and elevated sedimentation rate commonly seen

- **■ Differential Diagnosis**
  - Acute rheumatic fever
  - Juvenile rheumatoid arthritis
  - Viral exanthems
  - Infectious mononucleosis
  - Streptococcal pharyngitis

- **■ Treatment**
  - Intravenous immune globulin and high-dose aspirin are the mainstays of therapy
  - In carefully selected patients, bypass surgery if cardiac catheterization shows evidence of obstruction

Bacterial Meningitis

- ■ Essentials of Diagnosis
  - Signs of systemic illness (fever, malaise), headache, stiff neck, and altered mental status
  - In very young infants, signs of meningeal irritation may be absent
  - Predisposing factors include ear infection, sinusitis, immunodeficiencies, and recent neurosurgical procedures
  - No specific symptoms or signs reliably distinguish bacterial meningitis from meningitis due to viruses, fungi, or other pathogens
  - The causative organisms depends upon the age of the patient: < 1 month, group B or D streptococci, Enterobacteriaceae, *Listeria;* 1–3 months, above pathogens plus *Haemophilus influenzae,* pneumococci, and meningococci; 3 months to 7 years, *H influenzae,* pneumococci, and meningococci
  - Cerebrospinal fluid typically shows elevated protein, low glucose, high proportion of PMNs
  - Gram stain and culture often lead to the definitive diagnosis

- ■ Differential Diagnosis
  - Meningitis due to nonbacterial organisms
  - Brain abscess
  - Encephalitis
  - Sepsis without meningitis

- ■ Treatment
  - Prompt empiric antibiotics can be life-saving
  - Exact antibiotic regimen depends upon age of patient; therapy should be narrowed once the susceptibilities of the organism becomes known
  - Concomitant dexamethasone has been shown to decrease morbidity and mortality

17

Henoch-Schönlein Purpura (Anaphylactoid Purpura)

- **Essentials of Diagnosis**
    - A small-vessel vasculitis primarily affecting the skin, gastrointestinal tract, and kidney
    - Occurs primarily in males and most commonly in those 2–7 years of age; two-thirds have a preceding upper respiratory tract infection; occasionally observed in adults
    - The skin lesions often begin as urticaria and then progress to a macular-papular eruption which finally becomes a symmetric purpuric rash
    - Two-thirds of patients develop migratory polyarthralgias or polyarthritis; edema of the hands, feet, scalp, and periorbital areas occurs commonly
    - Abdominal pain, colicky in nature, is seen in half of patients; renal involvement is present in 25–50%
    - Platelet count, prothrombin time, and partial thromboplastin time are normal; urinalysis often reveals hematuria and proteinuria; serum IgA often elevated

- **Differential Diagnosis**
    - Immune thrombocytopenic purpura
    - Meningococcemia
    - Other hypersensitivity vasculitides
    - Juvenile rheumatoid arthritis
    - Kawasaki disease
    - Child abuse

- **Treatment**
    - Corticosteroid therapy may provide symptomatic relief but does not alter skin or renal manifestations
    - No satisfactory treatment
    - Prognosis is generally good

17

Croup Syndrome

- ## Essentials of Diagnosis
  - A group of diseases all leading to acute stridor; the clinical manifestations and treatment depend upon the specific disease
  - Viral croup, usually due to parainfluenza virus, affects younger children; a barking cough and stridor usually follow upper respiratory infection; high fever and drooling are absent
  - Epiglottitis is usually caused by *Haemophilus influenzae* type B and is characterized by sudden onset of fever, dysphagia, drooling, muffled voice, cyanosis, and soft stridor
  - Bacterial tracheitis (pseudomembranous croup), usually due to *Staphylococcus aureus,* represents localized mucosal invasion of bacteria in patients with viral croup; seen in patients with viral croup who deteriorate and develop high fever, toxicity, and upper airway obstruction
  - Lateral neck films can be useful diagnostically: patients with viral croup have subglottic narrowing and a normal epiglottis; those with epiglottitis have the classic "thumbprint" sign representing a swollen epiglottis; patients with bacterial tracheitis show a normal epiglottis but often have severe subglottic and tracheal narrowing
  - Direct laryngoscopy is very useful to rule out epiglottitis in confusing cases, but it must be performed cautiously with anticipation of intubation

- ## Differential Diagnosis
  - Spasmodic croup
  - Angioneurotic edema
  - Foreign body in the esophagus or larynx
  - Retropharyngeal abscess

- ## Treatment
  - Treatment of viral croup is supportive; mist therapy, oral hydration, oxygen, racemic epinephrine, and corticosteroids useful in some patients
  - Patients with epiglottitis require endotracheal intubation and intravenous antibiotics that cover *H influenzae*
  - Patients with bacterial tracheitis should be treated like those with epiglottitis except that the antibiotic chosen should also cover *S aureus*

17

Hemolytic-Uremic Syndrome

- ■ Essentials of Diagnosis
  - The most common single cause of renal failure due to glomerular vascular injury in children
  - Characterized by the triad of hemolytic anemia, thrombocytopenia, and renal failure
  - Primary lesion is to the endothelium of the arterioles, especially in the kidney, with formation of platelet thrombi
  - Cause is unknown but may involve both a genetic and an infectious or immunologic component; toxigenic *E. coli* (0157:H7) in some cases
  - Most often seen in children less than 2 years of age; older children have a more severe course and worse prognosis
  - Usually begins with a prodromal phase characterized by diarrhea, abdominal pain, and vomiting

- ■ Differential Diagnosis
  - Acute glomerulonephritis
  - Disseminated intravascular coagulation (DIC)
  - Immune thrombocytopenic purpura
  - Acute tubular necrosis
  - Hemolysis due to other causes

- ■ Treatment
  - Early dialysis and strict attention to fluid and electrolyte balance
  - Plasma infusion of plasmapharesis in severe cases
  - Red cell and platelet transfusions as needed for bleeding
  - Most children recover completely

18

Common Disorders of the Eye

Acute Conjunctivitis

- **Essentials of Diagnosis**
  - Acute onset of red, itchy, painful eyes with tearing and discharge
  - Conjunctival and peripheral scleral injection with or without preauricular lymph node enlargement
  - Vision is normal
  - Causes include bacterial, chlamydial, and viral infections, allergy, chemical irritation, and keratoconjunctivitis sicca

- **Differential Diagnosis**
  - Acute uveitis
  - Acute glaucoma
  - Corneal trauma or infection

- **Treatment**
  - Topical ophthalmologic antibiotics
  - Ophthalmology follow-up for persistent symptoms or presence of decreased visual acuity

Corneal Ulceration

- ■ Essentials of Diagnosis
  - Acute eye pain, photophobia, redness, tearing, blurred vision
  - Conjunctival and circumcorneal scleral injection; corneal defect by slitlamp examination and fluorescein dye
  - Causes include trauma, infection (bacterial, herpetic, fungal, *Acanthamoeba*)

- ■ Differential Diagnosis
  - Acute uveitis
  - Acute glaucoma
  - Acute conjunctivitis

- ■ Treatment
  - Topical antibiotics, patching of eye for 24 hours, and early ophthalmologic follow-up
  - Prompt ophthalmologic referral if infective cause is suspected

Acute (Angle-Closure) Glaucoma

- ■ Essentials of Diagnosis
  - Five percent of all glaucoma
  - Acute onset of eye pain, photophobia, blurred vision with halos around lights, headaches, nausea, abdominal pain
  - Conjunctival and circumcorneal scleral injection, steamy cornea, pupil mildly dilated and nonreactive; elevated intraocular pressure by tonometry
  - Preexisting narrow anterior chamber angle predisposes; elderly, hyperopes, Asians more susceptible; precipitated by pupillary dilation—stress, pharmacologic mydriasis (ophthalmologic examination or systemic anticholinergic use), dark environment

- ■ Differential Diagnosis
  - Acute conjunctivitis
  - Acute uveitis
  - Corneal trauma or infection

- ■ Treatment
  - Prompt ophthalmologic referral
  - Lower intraocular pressure with acetazolamide, osmotic diuresis, and topical pilocarpine
  - Laser peripheral iridectomy usually curative

18

Open-Angle (Chronic) Glaucoma

- **Essentials of Diagnosis**
  - Insidious onset of loss of peripheral vision ending with tunnel vision; asymptomatic early; common in blacks
  - Tonometry reveals persistent elevation of intraocular pressure; pathologic cupping of optic disk seen funduscopically
  - Loss of peripheral vision by peripheral fields

- **Differential Diagnosis**
  - Diurnal elevation (normal) of intraocular pressure
  - Bilateral retinal disorders (diabetic retinopathy, senile macular degeneration)

- **Treatment**
  - Timolol (beta-adrenergic blocking agent)
  - Miotics (pilocarpine)
  - Epinephrine ophthalmologic drops
  - Carbonic anhydrase inhibitors
  - Laser trabeculoplasty and surgical trabeculectomy are being increasingly used

Uveitis

- ■ **Essentials of Diagnosis**
  - Defined as inflammation of the uveal tract, which consists of the iris (iritis), ciliary body (cyclitis), and choroid (choroiditis)
  - Rapid onset of unilateral eye pain, photophobia, blurred vision or visual loss (anterior); gradual visual loss but otherwise asymptomatic (posterior)
  - Injected circumcorneal sclera with flare and inflammatory cells by examination of anterior chamber (anterior uveitis) or vitreous (posterior uveitis) or both (panuveitis) by slitlamp examination
  - Multiple causes associated: HLA B27-associated autoimmune disease (eg, ankylosing spondylitis, Reiter's syndrome, ulcerative colitis), Behçet's syndrome, infectious (herpes simplex or zoster, syphilis, toxoplasmosis, leprosy), sarcoidosis

- ■ **Differential Diagnosis**
  - Acute conjunctivitis
  - Corneal ulceration
  - Retinal detachment
  - Intraocular tumor
  - Multiple sclerosis

- ■ **Treatment**
  - Prompt ophthalmologic referral in all cases
  - Anterior disease: topical steroids, dilation of the pupil
  - Posterior disease: more commonly requires systemic steroids and immunosuppressants
  - Surveillance and treatment of underlying disease or cause is mandatory

18

Cataract

- ■ Essentials of Diagnosis
  - • Slowly progressive blurred vision without pain or other symptoms
  - • Lens opacities grossly visible or seen by ophthalmoscopy

- ■ Differential Diagnosis
  - • Generally unmistakable
  - • Ectopia lentis may cause some diagnostic confusion

- ■ Treatment
  - • Surgical removal for visual impairment or occupational requirement
  - • Subsequent intraocular lenses or soft contact lenses following surgery

Central Retinal Vein Occlusion

■ **Essentials of Diagnosis**
- Variable visual loss, usually unilateral upon awakening
- Disk edema, venous dilation or tortuosity, retinal hemorrhage or cotton wool spots by funduscopy
- Branch retinal vein occlusion associated with Behçet's syndrome

■ **Differential Diagnosis**
- Macular depression
- Central retinal artery occlusion
- Chronic glaucoma
- Vitreal hemorrhage
- Retinal detachment

■ **Treatment**
- Prompt ophthalmologic referral
- Surveillance for underlying diabetes, hyperlipidemia, hypertension, hyperviscosity syndrome (eg, Waldenström's macroglobulinemia)

Central Retinal Artery Occlusion

- ■ Essentials of Diagnosis
    - Sudden painless visual loss, usually severe (central)
    - Pallid edematous retina, cherry-red spot at the fovea reflecting maintained external carotid circulation
    - Associated underlying diseases include giant cell arteritis, cardiac or aortic emboli, migraine, oral contraceptives, antiphospholipid antibody syndromes

- ■ Differential Diagnosis
    - Vitreal hemorrhage
    - Retinal detachment
    - Central retinal vein occlusion
    - Acute glaucoma
    - Ocular migraine

- ■ Treatment
    - Medical emergency calling for immediate ophthalmologic referral
    - Patient to lie still, supine; ocular massage, supplemental oxygen, intravenous acetazolamide, anterior chamber paracentesis

Retinal Detachment

- ■ Essentials of Diagnosis
  - Painless, blurred vision in one eye which is progressive ("curtain closing over visual field")
  - Detachment seen by ophthalmoscopy
  - Cataract extraction and myopia predispose

- ■ Differential Diagnosis
  - Vitreous hemorrhage
  - Occlusion of central artery or retinal vein

- ■ Treatment
  - Immediate ophthalmologic referral in all cases
  - Placement of patient's head so that gravity will reposition retina
  - Closure of retinal tear by cryosurgery, scleral buckling, or both
  - Repair of small tears by photocoagulation

18

19

Common Disorders of the Ear, Nose, & Throat

Chronic Serous Otitis Media

- **Essentials of Diagnosis**
  - Due to blockage of the auditory (eustachian) tube, resulting in transudation of fluid
  - More common in children but can occur in adults following an upper respiratory tract infection, barotrauma, or auditory tube obstruction by tumor
  - Painless hearing loss with feeling of fullness or voice reverberation in affected ear
  - Dull, immobile tympanic membrane with loss of landmarks; intact light reflex
  - Fifteen- to twenty-decibel conductive hearing loss by audiometry

- **Differential Diagnosis**
  - Acute otitis media
  - Nasopharyngeal tumor (as causative agent)

- **Treatment**
  - Oral decongestants and antihistamines
  - Tympanotomy tubes for refractory cases with otolaryngologic referral
  - Inhaled nasal steroids also helpful

Acute Otitis Media

- **Essentials of Diagnosis**
  - Ear pain, with sensation of fullness in ear and hearing loss; fever and chills; onset often following upper respiratory syndrome
  - Dullness and hyperemia of eardrum with loss of landmarks and light reflex
  - Most common organisms in both children and adults include *Streptococcus pneumoniae, Haemophilus influenzae,* and *Streptococcus pyogenes*
  - Complications include mastoiditis, skull base osteomyelitis, sigmoid sinus thromboses, meningitis, brain abscess

- **Differential Diagnosis**
  - Bullous myringitis
  - Acute external otitis
  - Otalgia referred from other sources
  - Serous otitis

- **Treatment**
  - Antibiotics (controversial) and oral decongestants
  - Myringotomy if infection does not resolve or if hearing loss or vertigo develops or for recurrent infections
  - Recurrent acute otitis media may be prevented with long-term antibiotic prophylaxis

19

Endolymphatic Hydrops (Meniere's Syndrome)

- ■ Essentials of Diagnosis
  - Due to distention of the endolymphatic compartment of the inner ear
  - Episodic vertigo and nausea (lasting 1–8 hours) with oral pressure; low tone tinnitus
  - Progressive sensorineural hearing loss by audiometry
  - Causes include recent or remote head trauma and syphilis

- ■ Differential Diagnosis
  - Positioning vertigo
  - Posterior fossa tumor
  - Vestibular neuronitis
  - Vertebrobasilar insufficiency
  - Psychiatric disorder
  - Multiple sclerosis

- ■ Treatment
  - Low-salt diet and diuretic
  - Antihistamines, diazepam, and antiemetics may be given parenterally for acute attacks
  - Surgical decompression of endolymphatic sac for refractory cases

Benign Positioning Vertigo

- ■ Essentials of Diagnosis
  - Acute onset of vertigo, nausea, tinnitus
  - Provoked by changes in head positioning rather than by maintenance of a particular posture
  - Nystagmus with positive Bárány test (delayed onset of symptoms by movement of head with habituation and fatigue of symptoms)

- ■ Differential Diagnosis
  - Endolymphatic hydrops
  - Vestibular neuronitis
  - Posterior fossa tumor
  - Vertebrobasilar insufficiency

- ■ Treatment
  - Intravenous diazepam, antihistamines, and antiemetics for acute attack
  - Reassurance with otolaryngologic referral for persistent symptoms or other neurologic abnormalities
  - Single-session physical therapy protocols may be useful in some patients

Acute Sinusitis

- ■ Essentials of Diagnosis
  - Nasal congestion, purulent discharge, facial pain, and headache; teeth may hurt or feel abnormal in maxillary sinusitis; history of allergic rhinitis or acute upper respiratory or dental infection often present
  - Tenderness, erythema, and swelling over affected sinus; fever; discolored nasal discharge and poor response to decongestants alone
  - Clouding of sinuses on radiography or by transillumination
  - Coronal CT scans have become the diagnostic study of choice
  - Pain may not be prominent in chronic sinusitis
  - Typical pathogens include *Streptococcus pneumoniae,* other streptococci, *Haemophilus influenzae, Staphylococcus aureus,* and *Moraxella catarrhalis*

- ■ Differential Diagnosis
  - Viral or allergic rhinitis
  - Dental abscess
  - Dacryocystitis
  - Carcinoma of sinus
  - Headache due to other causes, especially cluster headache

- ■ Treatment
  - Oral and nasal decongestants, broad-spectrum antibiotics for acute cases with avoidance of sinus manipulation
  - Polypectomy, septal resection, or intranasal antrotomy for chronic disease

Allergic Rhinitis (Hay Fever)

- **■ Essentials of Diagnosis**
  - Seasonal or perennial occurrence of watery nasal discharge, sneezing, itching of eyes and nose
  - Pale, boggy mucous membranes with conjunctival injection
  - Eosinophilia of nasal secretions and occasionally of blood
  - Positive skin tests often present but of little value in most instances

- **■ Differential Diagnosis**
  - Upper respiratory viral infections

- **■ Treatment**
  - Desensitization occasionally beneficial
  - Oral antihistamines; oral or inhaled decongestants
  - Short-course systemic steroids for severe cases
  - Nasal corticosteroids and nasal cromolyn sodium often effective if used correctly

Epiglottitis

- **Essentials of Diagnosis**
  - Sudden onset of stridor, odynophagia, dysphagia, and drooling
  - Cherry-red, swollen epiglottis on indirect laryngoscopy; pharynx typically normal or slightly injected
  - Should be suspected when odynophagia is out of proportion to pharyngeal findings
  - Muffled voice, toxic-appearing and febrile patient

- **Differential Diagnosis**
  - Viral croup
  - Foreign body in larynx
  - Retropharyngeal abscess

- **Treatment**
  - Humidified oxygen with no manipulation of oropharynx or epiglottis
  - Intubation if necessary, preferably performed in an operating room with tracheostomy set available
  - Parenteral antibiotics active against *Haemophilus influenzae* and systemic corticosteroids

External Otitis (Swimmer's Ear)

- ■ Essentials of Diagnosis
  - Presents with otalgia, often accompanied by pruritus and purulent discharge
  - Usually caused by gram-negative rods or fungi
  - Often a history of water exposure or trauma to the ear canal
  - Movement of the auricle often produces pain; erythema and edema of the ear canal with a purulent exudate often noted on examination
  - Though the tympanic membrane is usually red, it moves normally with pneumatic otoscopy

- ■ Differential Diagnosis
  - Malignant otitis externa (persistent external otitis in an immuno-compromised or diabetic patient that evolves into osteomyelitis of the skull bone); *Pseudomonas* causative in diabetes

- ■ Treatment
  - Prevent additional moisture and mechanical injury to the ear canal
  - Otic drops containing a mixture of an aminoglycoside and a corticosteroid
  - Purulent debris filling the canal should be removed; occasionally a wick is needed to facilitate entry of the otic drops

19

Viral Rhinitis (Common Cold)

- **Essentials of Diagnosis**
  - Headache, nasal congestion, watery rhinorrhea, sneezing, scratchy throat, and malaise
  - Due to a variety of viruses, including rhinovirus and adenovirus
  - Examination of the nares reveals a reddened, erythematous mucosa and watery discharge

- **Differential Diagnosis**
  - Acute sinusitis
  - Allergic rhinitis
  - Bacterial pharyngitis

- **Treatment**
  - Supportive treatment only
  - Decongestants and phenylephrine nasal sprays (should not be used for more than 10 days) may be useful
  - Secondary bacterial infection is suggested by a change of rhinorrhea from clear to yellow or green; cultures are useful to guide antimicrobial therapy

20

Poisoning

Acetaminophen

- ■ Essentials of Diagnosis
  - Patients may develop nausea and vomiting after ingestion
  - Otherwise asymptomatic until 24–48 hours after ingestion
  - Serum acetaminophen levels should be measured upon initial evaluation and repeated at 4-hour intervals if any concern persists; a level should be obtained in all overdoses
  - All cases show striking elevations in aminotransferases; in some, fulminant hepatic necrosis may develop

- ■ Differential Diagnosis
  - Other hepatotoxin ingestion (eg, *Amanita* mushrooms, carbon tetrachloride)
  - Alcoholic liver disease
  - Viral hepatitis

- ■ Treatment
  - Activated charcoal as for all ingestions
  - Gastric lavage if less than 3–4 hours since ingestion
  - If serum acetaminophen level is higher than the toxic line on standard nomogram, administer acetylcysteine, 140 mg/kg orally, followed by 70 mg/kg every 4 hours

Amphetamines, Cocaine, Phencyclidine

- ■ Essentials of Diagnosis
  - Anxiety, tremulousness, tachycardia, hypertension, diaphoresis
  - Dilated pupils, agitation, muscular hyperactivity, psychosis, hyperthermia, seizures
  - Metabolic acidosis may occur
  - PCP: Vertical and horizontal nystagmus

- ■ Differential Diagnosis
  - Anticholinergic poisoning
  - Functional psychosis
  - Exertional heat stroke

- ■ Treatment
  - Activated charcoal as for all ingestions
  - Gastric lavage if less than 3–4 hours since ingestion
  - For hyperthermia, cooling with water sponge bath
  - For hypertension: phentolamine, nifedipine, nitroprusside, or labetalol
  - For arrhythmias, use esmolol, not propranolol (because unopposed alpha-adrenergic effects may worsen hypertension); short half-life of esmolol allows rapid dissipation of effect
  - For agitation or psychosis, sedation with benzodiazepines or neuroleptics

Anticholinergics

- **Essentials of Diagnosis**
  - Anticholinergic drugs include atropine (and diphenoxylate with atropine), scopolamine, tricyclic antidepressants, and antihistamines
  - Dry mouth, thirst, difficulty in swallowing, blurring of vision
  - Hyperthermia with absence of sweating
  - Dilated pupils, flushed skin, tachycardia, delirium, myoclonus, ileus, flushed appearance, seizures
  - Prolonged QT interval and torsade de pointes with newer nonsedating antihistamines

- **Differential Diagnosis**
  - Amphetamines or other stimulant overdose
  - LSD or other hallucinogen ingestion

- **Treatment**
  - Activated charcoal for all ingestions
  - Gastric lavage if less than 3–4 hours since ingestion
  - Supportive measures with cool water sponge bath for hyperthermia, sedation for agitation
  - Bicarbonate intravenously for tricyclic antidepressant-related cardiotoxicity

Arsenic

- **Essentials of Diagnosis**
  - Found in pesticides and industrial chemicals
  - Symptoms of poisoning usually appear within 1 hour after ingestion but may be delayed as long as 12 hours
  - Severe abdominal pain, vomiting, diarrhea, skeletal muscle cramps, dehydration, and shock in acute overdose
  - With chronic ingestion, hair loss, peripheral sensory neuropathy, anemia with basophilic stippling may occur

- **Differential Diagnosis**
  - Thallium toxicity
  - Other heavy metal toxicity

- **Treatment**
  - Activated charcoal as for all ingestions
  - Gastric lavage if less than 3–4 hours since ingestion
  - Dimercaprol (BAL) intramuscularly plus oral penicillamine for symptomatic patients or those with massive overdose

Beta-Blockers

- **Essentials of Diagnosis**
  - Hypotension, bradycardia, atrioventricular block
  - Seizures and coma may occur with propranolol and other lipid soluble agents
  - Hyperkalemia

- **Differential Diagnosis**
  - Tricyclic antidepressants
  - Calcium antagonist overdose
  - Digitalis intoxication

- **Treatment**
  - Activated charcoal as for all ingestions
  - Gastric lavage if less than 3–4 hours since ingestion
  - Supportive therapy for coma, hypotension, and seizures
  - Atropine, isoproterenol, or pacemaker for bradycardia or heart block
  - Glucagon for refractory bradycardia and hypotension

Calcium Antagonists (Calcium Channel Blockers)

- **Essentials of Diagnosis**
  - Bradycardia, atrioventricular block, hypotension
  - Arteriolar vasodilation and depression of cardiac contractility
  - Cardiac arrest with severe poisoning

- **Differential Diagnosis**
  - Beta-blocker overdose or toxicity
  - Tricyclic antidepressant overdose or toxicity
  - Digitalis overdose or toxicity

- **Treatment**
  - Activated charcoal as for all ingestions
  - Gastric lavage if less than 3–4 hours since ingestion
  - Supportive therapy for coma, hypotension, and seizures
  - Intravenous calcium chloride or calcium gluconate to reverse negative inotropic effects
  - Epinephrine infusion and intravenous glucagon may be helpful
  - Pacemaker as needed for bradycardia or heart block

Carbon Monoxide

■ Essentials of Diagnosis

- Colorless, odorless gas produced by the combustion of carbon-containing materials
- Poisoning may result from exposure to automobile exhaust, smoke inhalation, or accidental exposure to an improperly vented gas heater or other appliance
- Symptoms include headache, dizziness, abdominal pain, nausea, flushed skin, altered mentation
- Confusion, dyspnea, syncope, hypotension, coma, and seizures may develop in severe poisoning
- Survivors of severe poisoning may have permanent neurologic deficits
- Elevated arterial or venous carboxyhemoglobin level; blood gas testing yields falsely normal calculated oxyhemoglobin saturation

■ Differential Diagnosis

- Cyanide poisoning
- Depressant drug ingestion
- In chronic intoxication, headache of other cause

■ Treatment

- Remove from exposure
- Maintain airway and assist ventilation as necessary
- 100% oxygen
- Hyperbaric oxygen for patients with coma or seizures and in pregnant women

Cardiac Glycosides (Digitalis)

- ■ Essentials of Diagnosis
  - Intoxication may result from acute single exposure or chronic accidental overmedication
  - Acute overdose: nausea, vomiting, severe hyperkalemia, visual disturbances, bradycardia, atrioventricular block
  - Chronic toxicity: nausea, vomiting, xanthopsia, ventricular arrhythmias
  - Elevated serum digoxin level in acute overdose; level may be normal with chronic toxicity

- ■ Differential Diagnosis
  - Beta-blocker effect or toxicity
  - Calcium blocker effect or toxicity
  - Tricyclic antidepressants toxicity

- ■ Treatment
  - Activated charcoal as for all ingestions
  - Gastric lavage if less than 3–4 hours since ingestion
  - Maintain adequate airway and assist ventilation as necessary
  - Correct hyperkalemia or hypokalemia. (*Caution:* Do not give calcium.)
  - Lidocaine or phenytoin for ventricular arrhythmias
  - Atropine, isoproterenol, pacemaker for bradycardia, atrioventricular block
  - Digoxin antibodies for refractory arrhythmias, hypotension, hyperkalemia

Cyanide

- **Essentials of Diagnosis**
    - Toxic chemical used in research and commercial laboratories; important component of smoke in fires; also generated by the breakdown of nitroprusside
    - Instantaneous onset of symptoms including headache, dizziness, nausea, abdominal pain, anxiety, hyperventilation, altered mentation
    - Severe poisoning may result in syncope, shock, hypotension, apnea, seizures, coma, and death
    - Odor of almonds may be present on patient's breath or in vomitus
    - Venous oxygen saturation may be elevated because tissues have failed to take up arterial oxygen

- **Differential Diagnosis**
    - Carbon monoxide poisoning
    - Hydrogen sulfide poisoning

- **Treatment**
    - Activated charcoal as for all ingestions
    - Gastric lavage if less than 3–4 hours since ingestion
    - Maintain adequate airway and assist ventilation as necessary
    - Supportive therapy for coma, hypotension, and seizures
    - Amyl or sodium nitrate plus sodium thiosulfate antidotes

Iron

- **Essentials of Diagnosis**
  - Corrosive to the gastrointestinal tract and has depressant effects on the myocardium and on peripheral vascular resistance
  - Vomiting (sometimes with hematemesis), diarrhea, hypotension, acidosis
  - Shock due to massive fluid losses, bleeding, acidosis, sepsis
  - Elevated serum iron levels
  - Radiopaque tablets may be visible on plain abdominal radiographs

- **Differential Diagnosis**
  - Other heavy metal toxicity
  - Salicylate overdose
  - Theophylline overdose

- **Treatment**
  - Activated charcoal is not effective but should be used if other ingestants suspected
  - Gastric lavage if less than 3–4 hours since ingestion
  - Whole bowel irrigation, endoscopic or surgical removal if tablets visible on abdominal radiograph
  - Aggressive intravenous fluid and pressor support
  - Parenteral deferoxamine for chelation

Isoniazid (INH)

- ■ Essentials of Diagnosis
  - Confusion, slurred speech, seizures with acute overdose
  - Severe lactic acidosis due to inhibited metabolism of lactate
  - Hepatic toxicity with chronic use in certain patients

- ■ Differential Diagnosis
  - Convulsions due to other causes, eg, other convulsant drugs
  - Hepatitis of other cause

- ■ Treatment
  - Activated charcoal as for all ingestions
  - Gastric lavage if less than 3–4 hours since ingestion
  - Maintain adequate airway and assist ventilation as necessary
  - Supportive therapy for coma, hypotension, and seizures
  - Intravenous diazepam for seizures
  - Pyridoxine (vitamin B_6) as an antidote for seizures that do not respond to diazepam

Lead

- ## Essentials of Diagnosis
  - Lead toxicity usually results from chronic, repeated exposure
  - Colicky abdominal pain, constipation, headache, irritability, learning disorders in children, motor neuropathy
  - Coma or seizures with severe poisoning
  - Microcytic anemia with basophilic stippling
  - Blood lead level > 50 μg/dL, elevated free erythrocyte protoporphyrin

- ## Differential Diagnosis
  - Other heavy metal toxicity
  - Porphyria

- ## Treatment
  - Remove patient from exposure
  - Maintain adequate airway and assist ventilation as necessary
  - Supportive therapy for coma and seizures
  - Whole bowel irrigation, endoscopy, or surgical removal if large lead-containing object visible in the stomach on abdominal radiograph
  - Chelation with intravenous calcium EDTA with or without intramuscular dimercaprol if patient is encephalopathic
  - Dimercaptosuccinic acid (DMSA) for oral use in patients with mild to moderate intoxication
  - Investigate source and test other workers or family members who might have been exposed

Lithium

- ■ Essentials of Diagnosis
  - Ataxia, polyuria, delirium, coma, seizures
  - Dehydration, tremor, rigidity
  - Elevated serum lithium (> 2.0 meq/L); leukocytosis with neutrophilia, a common effect of lithium
  - Nephrogenic diabetes insipidus often complicates

- ■ Differential Diagnosis
  - Other psychotropic drug intoxication
  - Neuroleptic malignant syndrome

- ■ Treatment
  - Activated charcoal as for all ingestions
  - Gastric lavage if less than 3–4 hours since ingestion
  - Close management of volume and electrolytes
  - Hydration with normal saline
  - Hemodialysis for severely symptomatic patients

Methanol & Ethylene Glycol

- **Essentials of Diagnosis**
  - Methanol is found in solvents, duplicating fluids, record cleaning solutions, and paint removers; ethylene glycol is found in antifreeze
  - Symptoms include inebriation, lethargy, coma, seizures
  - Elevated serum osmolality and osmolar gap occur initially
  - After several hours, an anion gap metabolic acidosis occurs with tachypnea, confusion, and progression to seizures, coma
  - Visual disturbances with methanol; oxalate crystalluria and renal failure with ethylene glycol
  - Urine may fluoresce under a Wood lamp in ethylene glycol ingestions if fluorescein was added to the ethylene glycol product

- **Differential Diagnosis**
  - Other anion gas acidosis
  - Other alcohol (eg, ethanol, isopropanol) ingestions
  - Salicylate overdose

- **Treatment**
  - Activated charcoal as for all ingestions
  - Gastric lavage if less than 3–4 hours since ingestion
  - Maintain adequate airway and assist ventilation as necessary
  - Supportive therapy for coma and seizures
  - Sodium bicarbonate in presence of metabolic acidosis to enhance excretion of toxic acids
  - Ethanol infusion to level of 100 mg/dL
  - Hemodialysis for severe toxicity

Methemoglobinemia

- **Essentials of Diagnosis**
    - Drugs that can oxidize ferrous hemoglobin to its ferric state (methemoglobin) include benzocaine, aniline, nitrites, nitrogen oxide gases, dapsone, and pyridium
    - Symptoms of methemoglobinemia include dizziness, nausea, headache, dyspnea, altered mentation, seizures, coma
    - Cyanosis with normal P_{O_2} by arterial blood gas measurement
    - Inaccurate pulse oximetry measurements; decreased oxyhemoglobin saturation (usually about 85%) by arterial blood gas measurement
    - Blood may appear chocolate brown color
    - Hemolysis may occur in patients susceptible to oxidant stress (eg, G6PD deficiency)

- **Differential Diagnosis**
    - Hypoxia or ischemia
    - Sulfhemoglobinemia
    - Carbon monoxide poisoning

- **Treatment**
    - Activated charcoal for recent ingestions; repeat-dose charcoal for dapsone
    - Gastric lavage if less than 3–4 hours since ingestion
    - Discontinue offending agent
    - Oxygen; supportive therapy for coma and seizures
    - Maintain adequate airway and assist ventilation as necessary
    - Intravenous methylene for symptomatic patients with high levels

Opioids

- **Essentials of Diagnosis**
  - Somnolence, slurred speech, ataxia, coma, respiratory depression
  - Hypotension, bradycardia, hypothermia, hyporeflexia, pinpoint pupils
  - Pulmonary edema may occur
  - Signs of intravenous drug abuse

- **Differential Diagnosis**
  - Alcohol or sedative-hypnotic overdose
  - Clonidine overdose
  - Phenothiazine overdose
  - Congestive heart failure
  - Infectious or metabolic encephalopathy

- **Treatment**
  - Activated charcoal as for all ingestions
  - Gastric lavage if less than 3–4 hours since ingestion
  - Maintain adequate airway and assist ventilation as necessary
  - Supportive therapy for coma, hypothermia, and hypotension
  - Naloxone (duration 2–3 hours) for suspected overdose; repeat dosing as needed, or intravenous drip

Organophosphates

- **Essentials of Diagnosis**
  - Commonly used in pesticides, organophosphates cause an increase in acetylcholine activity at nicotinic and muscarinic receptors in the central nervous system
  - Abdominal cramps, excessive salivation, sweating, vomiting, diarrhea, lacrimation, pinpoint pupils
  - Wheezing, bronchorrhea, fasciculations, seizures, skeletal muscle weakness
  - Tachycardia followed by bradycardia
  - Serum and red blood cell cholinesterase activity depressed

- **Differential Diagnosis**
  - Carbamate (insecticide) poisoning
  - Curare or neuromuscular blocker poisoning

- **Treatment**
  - Activated charcoal as for all ingestions
  - Gastric lavage if less than 3–4 hours since ingestion
  - If agent is on the victim's skin or hair, wash repeatedly with soap or shampoo and water
  - Give oxygen; maintain adequate airway and assist ventilation as necessary
  - Atropine, often needed in very large repeated doses
  - Pralidoxime (2-PAM) to reverse organophosphate binding

Salicylates

- ■ **Essentials of Diagnosis**
    - Acute ingestion: Nausea, vomiting, gastritis
    - Moderate intoxication: Hyperpnea, tachycardia, tinnitus, elevated anion gap metabolic acidosis
    - Severe intoxication: Agitation, confusion, coma, seizures, cardiovascular collapse, pulmonary edema, hyperthermia, hypoprothrombinemia, hypoglycemia
    - Metabolic acidosis, respiratory alkalosis
    - Elevated serum salicylate level

- ■ **Differential Diagnosis**
    - Carbon monoxide poisoning
    - Methanol or ethylene glycol ingestion

- ■ **Treatment**
    - Activated charcoal as for all ingestions
    - Gastric lavage if less than 3–4 hours since ingestion
    - Maintain adequate airway and assist ventilation as necessary
    - Supportive therapy for coma, hyperthermia, hypotension, and seizures
    - Intravenous fluid therapy with alkalinization of the urine enhances salicylate excretion
    - Hemodialysis for severe metabolic acidosis, markedly altered mental status, or significantly elevated salicylate levels after acute overdose

Sedative-Hypnotics

- ■ Essentials of Diagnosis
  - Euphoria, slurred speech, ataxia
  - Stupor, coma, and respiratory arrest in severe cases
  - Hypotension, bradycardia, hypothermia, hyporeflexia
  - Pulmonary edema may occur with severe overdose

- ■ Differential Diagnosis
  - Opioid overdose
  - Medical disease of central nervous system (eg, encephalitis)
  - Metabolic encephalopathy

- ■ Treatment
  - Activated charcoal as for all ingestions
  - Gastric lavage if less than 3–4 hours since ingestion
  - Maintain adequate airway and assist ventilation as necessary
  - Supportive therapy for coma, hypotension, and hypothermia
  - Flumazenil for severe benzodiazepine intoxication; precipitation of seizures possible if patient is a habitual user
  - Repeat-dose charcoal and hemoperfusion for severe phenobarbital intoxications

Theophylline

- **Essentials of Diagnosis**
  - Mild intoxication: nausea, vomiting, tachycardia, tremulousness
  - Severe intoxication: tachyarrhythmias, hypotension, seizures
  - Acute overdose: hypokalemia, hyperglycemia, metabolic acidosis
  - Chronic intoxication: normal potassium and bicarbonate
  - Elevated serum theophylline level

- **Differential Diagnosis**
  - Caffeine overdose
  - Iron toxicity

- **Treatment**
  - Activated charcoal as for all ingestions; repeat doses may enhance theophylline elimination
  - Gastric lavage if less than 3–4 hours since ingestion
  - Oxygen; maintain adequate airway and assist ventilation as necessary
  - Treat seizures with diazepam and phenobarbital
  - Hemoperfusion for patients with status epilepticus or markedly elevated serum theophylline levels (> 100 µg/mL after acute overdose or > 60 µg/mL with chronic intoxication)
  - Esmolol for hypotension and tachycardia

Index

NOTE: Page numbers in **bold-face** indicate major discussions.